DERMATOLOGY QUICK GLANCE

NOTICE

DERMATOLOGY QUICK GLANCE

SAEED N. JAFFER, MD
Assistant Clinical Professor
UCLA School of Medicine
Los Angeles, California

ABRAR A. QURESHI, MD, MPH
Instructor in Dermatology
Harvard Medical School
Boston, Massachusetts

Foreword by Richard Allen Johnson, MDCM

McGraw-Hill
MEDICAL PUBLISHING DIVISION

New York Chicago San Francisco Lisbon
London Madrid Mexico City Milan New Delhi
San Juan Seoul Singapore Sydney Toronto

The McGraw·Hill Companies

DERMATOLOGY QUICK GLANCE

1 2 3 4 5 6 7 8 9 0 DOCDOC 0 9 8 7 6 5 4 3

ISBN 0-07-141526-2

This book was set in Times Roman by Westchester Book Group.
The editors were Darlene Cooke, Andrea Seils, Lisa Silverman, and Lester Sheinis.
The production supervisor was Richard C. Ruzycka.
The cover designer was Aimee Nordin.
The indexer was Alexandra Nickerson.
RR Donnelley was printer and binder.

This book is printed on acid-free paper.

Cataloging-in-Publication Data for this title is on file at the Library of Congress.

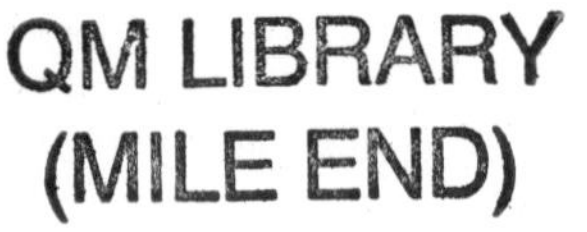

To my life partner, Kishwar, my children, Laila and Jamal,
and my pillars of support, Aboo, Mom, and Tehmina.
—Saeed

In loving memory of my late father, Aleem, my mother,
Kulsum, my wife, Laura, and our children, Afnaan and Danish.
—Abrar

CONTENTS

FOREWORD

The value of the printed word, whether in books or journals, has evolved greatly during the past decade. A new edition of *Harrison's Principles of Internal Medicine* is published every three and a half years; the current edition is also available on the Internet, where it is updated daily. Full text articles published in medical journals can also be read on the Internet, often prior to publication. Search engines such as PubMed from the National Library of Medicine can gather references within a matter of seconds on limitless subjects.

What then is the value of a new book in dermatology in this era of electronic publishing? The old adage "A picture is worth a thousand words" certainly is true for dermatologic textbooks. *Dermatology Quick Glance* by Jaffer and Qureshi demonstrates that tables and lists can be worth a thousand words. This new dermatology textbook summarizes the entire discipline of dermatology in fewer than 300 pages, providing easy access to thousands of factoids. Drs. Jaffer and Qureshi have compiled the search for a thousand and one subjects, which we all may have had in our memory banks at one point but have quickly forgotten after board or recertification examinations.

Who will find *Dermatology Quick Glance* of value? Individuals at the beginning a their careers, medical students, dermatology residents, and those studying for Dermatology Board Examinations and recertification. The book is also informative to leaf through, providing new associations, both new and/or forgotten. This presentation of factoids we hope will be updated in subsequent editions.

Richard Allen Johnson, MDCM

PREFACE

Dermatology Quick Glance is our collection of teaching materials and practical tidbits gathered over the years at the Boston area teaching hospitals affiliated with the medical schools of Harvard University, Boston University, and Tufts University.

For all those primary care providers on the front lines: you are aware that skin problems make up more than one-third of patient complaints. This book was written to help answer questions at the point of care and make dermatology as much fun and as exciting as we know it to be. It is meant to serve as a versatile, concise companion and to give providers that extra edge in providing complete care to their patients on a daily basis. It serves the needs of a wide audience:

- Medical students
- Residents and fellows of all specialties
- Nurse practitioners
- Physician assistants
- Nurses
- Emergency room physicians
- Family practitioners
- Pediatricians
- Internists

In particular, dermatology residents, dermatopathologists, and practicing dermatologists will use this book as a "peripheral brain" that allows rapid access both to simple facts and in-depth information. The format makes the book's contents readily accessible; it should prove functional in both a clinical environment and in studying for board examinations.

There is no one dermatology text like this one. The book is divided into 12 chapters that cover major topics in alphabetical order. Two chapters, "Infections and Parasites" and "Dermatopharmacology," are subdivided to facilitate quick reference. The text includes useful tables, illustrations, and flowcharts to explain complicated ideas in a simple, easy-to-understand fashion. Because of the wide variety of sources behind each component, references have been left out for the sake of brevity. Standard dermatologic abbreviations are utilized to present the information in a succinct manner.

We hope that you will find this book to be a valuable resource and guide. We will continue to strive to update and improve the information presented herein.

ACKNOWLEDGMENTS

There is one person who deserves more credit for the production of this work than any other: my wife, Kishwar Bano, who stuck with me through the worst and best at MIT, Harvard, UCLA, Boston University, and Tufts University. Thank you also to the people who first opened my eyes to the wonderful world of medicine and dermatology: my father, Dr. Shahnawaz S. Jaffer, Dr. Harley Haynes, and Dr. Richard Johnson. None of this would have been possible without the guidance and motivation provided by my mother, Aqueela Jaffer, and my sister, Tehmina Jaffer. Thanks to all my colleagues who have inspired and educated me throughout the years: Dan Loo, Abrar Qureshi, Vandana Chatrath, Rana Shahab, Mehran Nowfar-rad, Vince Afsahi, and Soma Wali.

Saeed N. Jaffer

There are many people who have contributed to my training and teaching from the Aga Khan University and Harvard Medical School. I simply cannot thank everyone. Saeed has been a true friend, colleague, and coauthor. My late father, Dr. Aleem S. Qureshi, a dermatologist and educator, was my best friend. He would have been proud of this work. For my mother, Dr. Kulsum Aleem: I truly appreciate all you have done. This book would not have been possible without my lovely wife Laura's outstanding strength, courage, and patience. For my sister Jazibeh and brothers Wasif and Tabarak: thank you for being there. Dr. Ethan Lerner has been like a father to me; I am grateful that he believed in me at a time when few others did. Dr. Harley Haynes is a role model whom I will always aspire to be like but will probably never be. Dr. Michael Bigby: thank you for instilling in me the thirst to learn more about evidence-based medicine.

Abrar A. Qureshi

SPECIAL MENTION

It is rare when a mentor comes along who significantly changes the lives of many pupils and colleagues at the same time. Dr. Daniel Loo is such an individual. His untiring commitment to teaching is the main inspiration behind the completion of this text.

We should like to credit, acknowledge, and thank Dr. Loo for his teaching. Although almost everyone completing dermatology residency compiles a list of factoids for studying, Dr. Loo helped initiate this project by putting these down on paper. In fact, a number of mnemonics incorporated in this book have his stamp of ingenuity on them. Although the final product presented here is an altogether different version, we are indebted to Dr. Loo for his tremendous guidance and support.

Saeed and Abrar

DERMATOLOGY QUICK GLANCE

CHAPTER

1

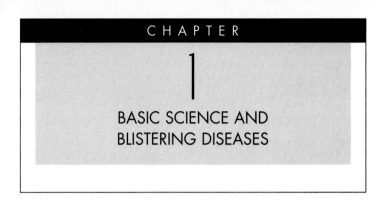

BASIC SCIENCE AND BLISTERING DISEASES

β-CATENIN

- Intracellular calcium-binding protein that is an "armadillo" protein (type of protein that permits cell-cell interaction)
- Increased expression in pilomatricoma
- Involved in morphogenesis of hair follicle
- Accumulates in stem cells
- Localizes to nucleus in melanoma

TABLE 1–1
AMINO ACIDS

Amino Acid	Fiber
Isodesmosine	Elastin
Desmosine	Elastin
Citrulline	Vimentin
Hydroxylysine	Collagen
Hydroxyproline	

TABLE 1–2
BLISTERING DISORDERS (AUTOIMMUNE)

Disease	Antigen	kDa	DIF	IIF	Salt Split
Pemphigoid (BP)	BPAG1 (less) BPAG2 (NC16 only)	230 180	100% linear C3 at BMZ; most also IgG	75% IgG1, IgG4 at BMZ Titer no help	Roof; 20% roof and base
Protein 105 pemphigoid	105-kDa protein in lower lamina lucida	105	Linear IgG at DEJ		All on the base
Cicatricial pemphigoid (CP)	Laminin 5 Laminin 6 BPAG1 BPAG2 (NC16 and collagenous domain)	150, 140 200 230 180 145/290	80+% linear IgG, C3 along BMZ, occasional IgM, IgA	20–30% IgG1, IgG4, IgA1	Roof or both or base only Laminin 5 or coll. VII
Ocular only	Collagen VII β_4 integrin	205			
Herpes gestationis (HG)	BPAG2 (NC16 only) BPAG1 (less)	180 230	100% linear C3 BMZ 40% IgG	25% IgG1 HG factor = identified by complement factor enhanced ELISA)	Roof
Pemphigus foliaceus	Desmoglein 1	160	100% IgG intercellular 50% C3	80–85% IgG4 guinea pig esophagus	
Pemphigus herpetiformis (neonatal)	Desmoglein 1 Desmoglein 3	160 130	100% IgG intercellular in upper or entire epidermis	Most have circulating IgG	

Pemphigus erythematosus (Senear-Usher disease)	Desmoglein 1	160	Intercellular IgG, C3 25% granular IgG, C3 at BMZ, 50% linear, positive lupus band	Circulating IgG Positive ANA
IgA pemphigus	Intraepidermal neutrophilic (IEN) desmoglein 3 Subcorneal pustular dermatosis (SPD) desmocollin 1 desmocollin 2	130 115 105	IEN: intercellular IgA1 in entire or lower epidermis SPD: intercellular IgA in upper epidermis only	50% have circulating IgA Skin culture best substrate
Pemphigus vulgaris	100% Dsg3 50–75% Dsg1	130 160	100% IgG intercellular 50% C3, IgA, IgM	80–85% IgG4 Best: monkey esophagus may follow titer
Paraneoplastic pemphigus	Plectin Desmoplakin I BPAG1 Desmoplakin II/envoplakin Periplakin Unknown Dsg1 Dsg3	500 250 230 210 190 170 160 130	Intercellular IgG, C3; may have linear C3 along BMZ	75–80% positive IgG on monkey esophagus Rodent bladder epithelium (best substrate)
Dermatitis herpetiformis	Transglutaminase (IgA antibodies)		100% granular IgA in papillary dermis	+Antigliadin Ab +Antiendomyseal Ab +Antireticulin Ab

TABLE 1–2
BLISTERING DISORDERS (AUTOIMMUNE) (*Continued*)

Disease	Antigen	kDa	DIF	IIF	Salt Split
Linear IgA disease Chronic bullous disease of childhood	LABD Ag (NC16 + coll. domain) LAD-1 (ladinin) Collagen VII	97/120 285 145/290	100% linear IgA BMZ on noninvolved skin	80%+ in children 30%+ in adults	Roof > both > base
EB acquisita	Collagen VII (noncollagenous)	145/290 dimer	100% linear IgG BMZ can be C3, IgM/A	25–50% IgG to BMZ	Floor
Bullous LE	Collagen VII (collagenous) Laminin 5 Laminin 6 BPAG1	145/290 dimer	100% linear IgG BMZ 50–60% linear IgA/M some C3	IgG, IgA when present	Floor, roof, or absent

Key: BMZ, basement membrane zone; DEJ, dermoepidermal junction; Ag, antigen; EB, epidermolysis bullosa; NC, noncollagenous.

BP230 and plectin homologous to desmoplakin 1.

97 kDa of LABD; Ag = extracellular domain of BPAg2 (180 kDa).

ELISA, enzyme-linked immunosorbent assay; NC16, noncollagenous domain of BP Ag2; NC domain collagen VII, fibronectin, von Willebrand factor, cartilage matrix protein; hemidesmosomes analogous to desmoplakin.

TABLE 1–3
BLISTERING DISORDERS (INHERITED VS. AUTOIMMUNE)

Antigen	Inherited Disorder	Autoimmune
K5, K14	EB[a] simplex	
Plectin	EB simplex–muscular dystrophy	Paraneoplastic pemphigus
BPAG2	Generalized atrophic benign EB (GABEB)	BP, HG, CP
α6β4 integrin	Junctional EB (JEB) with pulmonary atresia	β4 integrin: ocular CP only
Laminin V	JEB (occasional GABEB)	CP
Collagen VII	Dystrophic EB (collagenous domain)	Epidermolysis bullosa acquisita (noncollagenous domain), bullous lupus (collagenous domain)[a]

[a] EB = Epidermolysis bullosa.

[b] Transient bullous dermolysis of newborn heals spontaneously within months; may be dominant EB variant.

BLOTS

- Southern = DNA
- Northern = RNA
- Western = protein

CADHERINS

- Ca-dependent adhesion molecules
- Four types: E-cadherin, P-cadherin, desmoglein, desmocollin
- Cadherins present in both desmosomes and adherens junctions

TABLE 1–4
CD MARKERS

Cell Type	Associated With
CD1a+	Langerhans cells: histiocytosis X, Gianotti-Crosti syndrome
CD2, 3, 5, 7	Pan T cell, usually need fresh tissue
CD4+	Parapsoriasis, LyP type B, pityriasis lichenoides chronica (PLC)
CD4+, often CD7–, ↑CD4, ↓CD8	Cutaneous T-cell lymphoma (CTCL) • Mycosis fungoides
Th1	• Sézary syndrome
Th2	
CD8+	Pityriasis lichenoides et varioliformis acuta (PLEVA), lichen planus, graft-vs.-host disease, psoriasis, alopecia areata
CD8+	Actinic reticuloid
	Pagetoid reticulosis:
CD8+	• Local (Woringer-Kolopp disease)
CD4–, CD8–	• Disseminated (Ketron-Goodman disease)
CD10+	Folliculocentric B-cell lymphomas
CD15+, (may be CD30+)	Hodgkin disease
CD18	β_2-Integrin; defect = leukocyte adhesion deficiency type 1
CD20	Pan B-cell marker: ++ in B-cell lymphomas
CD21	Binds to EBV
CD25	Activated T cells (IL-2 receptor/Ontak® anti CD25 tagged with diptheria toxin)
CD30+	Lymphomatoid papulosis type A (type B = CD4+)
(Ki-1)	Large-cell anaplastic lymphoma (CTCL)
(Ber-H2)	Hodgkin disease
CD31	Endothelial cells, PECAM-1, angiosarcomas, Kaposi's sarcoma
C34+	Endothelials, DFSP (factor XIIIa-), Kaposi sarcoma, spindle cell lipoma
CD43	T cells, sialophorin (defect in Wiskott-Aldrich syndrome)
CD44	Extensive staining in Merkel cells indicates poor prognosis
CD45 (LCA)	White cells, Langerhans cells
CD45RO	Memory T cells
CD54	ICAM-1, which binds LFA-1
CD56	Natural killer (NK) cells (NK cell lympoma)
CD68+	Macrophages, JXG
CD79	Granulocytes, + myeloperoxidase, + chloracetate esterase = leukemia
CD95	Fas ligand (anti-Fas Ab used in toxic epidermal necrolysis) (Fas to ligand leads to apoptosis)
CD117	c-*kit* proto oncogene

COMMON LEUKOCYTE ANTIGEN MARKER (CLA)

- T cells that go to skin have CLA on their surfaces.
- Binds to E-selectin, located on endothelial cells in the skin's postcapillary venules.
- $\alpha_6\beta_7$ = marker for gut-homing T cells.

TABLE 1–5
COLLAGEN (TYPES AND DISTRIBUTION)

Collagen Type	Distribution	Disease
1	Skin, tendon, bone, deep dermis	Osteogenesis imperfecta, Ehlers-Danlos syndrome type VII
2	Cartilage	Relapsing polychondritis
3	Fetal skin, blood vessels, GI tract, papillary dermis	Ehlers-Danlos type IV (ecchymotic)
4	Basement membrane, lamina densa	Goodpasture syndrome, Alport syndrome; binds laminin via nidogen
5	Ubiquitous	Ehlers-Danlos types 1 + 2
6	Ubiquitous	
7	Anchoring fibrils, sublamina densa	Epidermolysis bullosa acquisita (EBA), dystrophic EB, bullous SLE; last BMZ part in embryo
8	Endothelial cells	"Like factor VIII"
9	Cartilage	
10	Cartilage	
11	Cartilage	
17	BPAG2, basement membrane zone Lamina lucida	Bullous pemphigoid (BP), cicatricial pemphigoid (CP), herpes gestationis (HG), paraneoplastic pemphigus (PNP), generalized atrophic benign EB (GABEB)

Collagen= 30% lysine, 10% proline.
Prolyl and Lysyl Hydroxylase need vitamin C.
Collagen has the following structure: Glycine-X-Y.
Collagen VII last component of basement membrane to appear in wound healing.

COMPLEMENT

- C5: complement for chemotaxis
- C3 common to both classic and alternative pathways
- ↓C3 = Partial lipodystrophy secondary C3 nephritic syndrome
- ↓C2, C4 = lupus
- ↓C5–C9 = susceptibility to disseminated *Neisseria* infections (asymptomatic urethritis, fever, arthritis, <12 acral pustules)
- ↓C1–C4 = susceptibility to SLE and glomerulonephritis

- ↓C1-INH = hereditary angioedema
- IgA stimulates alternative pathway
- C1 activated by antigen-bound IgM > IgG
- C3 activated (alternate pathway) in absence of antibody
- CH50: good measure of classic pathway

TABLE 1–6
CYTOKINES[a]

Cytokine	Cells	Characteristic Function
IFN-α_{2A}	Keratinocytes	Treat hemangioma, Kaposi sarcoma, malignant melanoma, mycosis fungoides
IFN-α_{2B}	Keratinocytes	Treat condyloma, Kaposi sarcoma, malignant melanoma, mycosis fungoides
IFN-γ	Activated T cells, NK cells	Th1, treat chronic granulomatous disease
IL-1	Keratinocytes	Fever in sunburn + gout; degranulates mast cells
IL-2	Activated T cells	Th1
IL-3	Mast cells	
IL-4	Mast cells, IgE isotype switching	Th2
IL-5	Mast cells, stimulate eosinophils	Th2
IL-6	B cells, keratinocytes	Jarisch-Herxheimer reaction
IL-8	Neutrophils	
IL-9	Mast cells, T cells	
IL-10	Keratinocytes	Th2, inhibitory
IL-12	Macrophages	Th1
IL-13	Mast cells, IgE isotype switching	Th2
TNF-α	Macrophages to migrate toward endothelium	Th1, Jarisch-Herxheimer reaction
TNF-β	Lymphotoxin	Th1
TGF-α	Keratinocytes, fibroblasts	Wound healing
TGF-β	Fibroblasts, Keratinocytes	Inhibitory

[a] See also Table 1–15, below.

TABLE 1–7
CONTENT OF ELASTIC FIBERS

Fibers	Fibrillin	Elastin
Oxytalan	⊕	↓
Elaunin	⊕	⊕
Elastic	↓	⊕

TABLE 1–8
EPIDERMOLYSIS BULLOSA (EB) MUTATIONS

EB	Gene	Mutation
EBS	*K5, K14* *Plectin*	• Koebner syndrome = generalized • Weber-Cockayne syndrome = palms/soles • Dowling-Meara syndrome = herpetiform • Muscular dystrophy
JEB	Laminin 5 chains: α_3 = *LAMA3* β_3 = *LAMB3* → 80% of mutations γ_2 = *LAMC2*	50% of β_3 mutations = R635X lead to Herlitz syndrome
DDEB	Collagen VII (*COL7A1*)	Missense spontaneous mutation → usually glycine substitution → → defective COL7A1 → defective anchoring fibrils → milder phenotype • Albopapuloid = atrophic white scars • Cockayne-Touraine syndrome = hyperplastic
RDEB	Collagen VII (*COL7A1*)	Double deletion mutations → incomplete COL7A1 → severe phenotype Hallopeau-Siemens type

Key: K, keratin; DDEB, dominant dystrophic EB; RDEB, recessive dystrophic EB.

TABLE 1–9
GENES

Oncogene	Features
ras	Small cell sarcoma, leukemia, sarcoma
jun	
RET	Extracellular domain defect (receptor): multiple endocrine neoplasia (MEN) type 2A Intracellular domain defect (kinase): MEN 2b (Sipple syndrome), Hirschsprung disease
myc	
fos	
bcl-2	Antiapoptotic (overexpressed in stem + basal cells) Protects melanocytes from UV-induced apoptosis (also nerve growth factor)
src	
sap	
smoothened	Basal cell carcinoma (BCC)[a]

TABLE 1–9
GENES (*Continued*)

Tumor Suppressor Gene	Features
p53	SCC, proapoptotic
Neurofibromin (chr. 17)	Neurofibromatosis-1 (suppresses *ras*)
Merlin (chr. 22)	Neurofibromatosis-2
Rb	Retinoblastoma
Tuberin (chr. 16)	Tuberous sclerosis (suppresses *ras*)
VHL	Von-Hippel–Lindau disease
APC	Familial polyposis coli + Gardner syndrome, APC = binds β-catenin
MTS-1	
PTEN	Cowden, Bannayan-Riley-Ruvalcalba syndrome, PTEN = phosphatase
Patched	Nevoid basal cell carcinoma syndrome (BCNS)
Patched mosaic	Nevus sebaceous
Hamartin (chr. 9)	Tuberous sclerosis
CDKN2A/ARF	Melanoma, familial pancreatic carcinoma
Serine threonine kinase (*STK11*)	Peutz-Jeghers syndrome

Other Genes	Features
hMSH2	DNA mismatch repair enzyme = Muir-Torre syndrome
Menin	Unknown mechanism for MEN type 1
ATM	Detects chromosome breaks, stops cell division = ataxia-telangiectasia
BLM	Helicase = Bloom syndrome
RECQL4	Helicase = Rothmund-Thomson syndrome
WRN	Helicase = Werner syndrome
HPV E5	Promotes epidermal proliferation
HPV E6	Inhibits *p53*
HPV E7	Inhibits *Rb*
Cyclid	Cylindroma
Fas	Proapoptotic

[a] Glutathione-*S*-transferase mutation leads to increased susceptibility to BCC.

HELICASE (RECQ) DEFECTS

- Werner syndrome (WRN gene)
- Bloom syndrome (BLM gene)
- Rothmund-Thomson syndrome (RECQL4)
- Cockayne syndrome = xeroderma pigmentosa type B
- Xeroderma pigmentosa type D = trichothiodystrophy

TABLE 1–10
HLA DISEASE ASSOCIATIONS

Disease	HLA Antigen
Fixed drug	B22
Lichen planus	DR10, DRw9, DR1, DR2
Psoriasis	DR406, Cw6
Psoriatic arthritis, Reiter syndrome	B27
Behçet disease	B51
Dermatitis herpetiformis (celiac disease)	DQw2, DR3, B8
Pemphigus vulgaris	Dw10, DR4
Herpes gestationis	DR3, DR4
Epidermolysis bullosa acquisita	DR2
Systemic lupus erythematosus (SLE)	Homozygous C4 + DR2 or DR3
Subacute cutaneous lupus erythematosus (SCLE)	DR3
Dermatomyositis	B8, DR3, DRw52, DQA1
Severe early alopecia areata	DR5
Sjögren syndrome	DR3

TABLE 1–11
SELECTED HUMAN LEUKOCYTE ANTIGENS IN NUMERICAL ORDER

Epidermolysis bullosa acquisita (EBA)	DR2
Collagen vascular disease	DR3
Pemphigus/bullous pemphigoid (BP)	DR4
Alopecia areata	DR5
Diabetes/dermatitis herpetiformis	B8
Lichen planus	DR10
Behçet syndrome	B51

INTERMEDIATE FILAMENTS = TONOFILAMENTS (8–10 nm)

- Keratins (epithelial cells)
- Vimentin (mesenchymal, including melanocytes)
- Desmin (muscle)
- Neurofilaments
- Nuclear laminins
- Nestin
- Glial fibrillary acid protein
- Peripherin

KERATINS

These make heptad units; defects occur in flanking regions/globular domains

Type 1 (smaller) (simple epithelium): acidic K10–K20, chromosome 17q
Type 2 (larger) (epidermis): basic K1–K9, chromosome 12q
Type 4 keratins = 1 protofilament
Type 2 protofilaments = 1 protofibril
Type 4 protofibrils = 1 keratin protofilament

TABLE 1–12
KERATINS

Keratin	Location	Disease	Clinical
1	Suprabasal	Unna-Thost palmoplantar keratoderma (PPK), monilethrix	
1, 10	Suprabasal	Epidermolytic hyperkeratosis (EHK) (bullous congenital ichthyosiform erythroderma)	Corrugated scale
2e	Late suprabasal/ granular layers	Ichthyosis bullosa of Siemens	Milder EHK
3, 12	Cornea	Corneal dystrophy of Messman	
4, 13	Mucosa	White sponge nevus of Canon	
5, 14	Basal layer	Epidermolysis bullosa (EB) simplex	3 types
5, 15	Mucosal basal layer		
6 6a, 16	Palmoplantar, mucosa, appendages (hyperproliferative states)	Monilethrix (6) + keratosis pilaris Pachyonychia congenita I (6a, 16)	Dystrophy, leukokeratosis
6b	Nail bed, myoepithelium		
17	Appendages/nail bed	Pachyonychia congenita II	Natal teeth, cysts
8, 18	Simple epithelium		
9	Palmoplantar	Epidermolytic PPK (Vorner)	
19	Bulge cells, simple epithelium		
20	Merkel cells	Merkel cell carcinoma	
21	Intestinal epithelium		
Plectin	Hemidesmosome + skeletal muscle	EB with muscular dystrophy	
α6β4 integrin	Hemidesmosome	Junctional EB with pyloric stenosis	

MACROPHAGE/MONOCYTE MARKERS

Monocyte-derived: MAC 387, HAM 56, lysozyme
Reactive: CD68

TABLE 1–13
MAST CELLS

Type	Enzyme	Location[a]
T type	Tryptase only	Bowel, respiratory mucosa
TC type	Tryptase + chymase	Skin, GI submucosa
C type	Chymase only	Skin, lymph nodes

[a] Systemic disease: Clinical = bone marrow (most common), diarrhea (give cromolyn), cramps, syncope. Test for serum tryptase level or methylimidazole, acetic acid, and methylhistamine increased in urine.

TABLE 1–14
MAST CELL MEDIATORS

Preformed		Newly Formed (released after IgE binding)	
Histamine	• Proteoglycans	Prostaglandin D2 (#1)	IL-4, IL-5, Il-6, IL-8
Heparin	Kininogenase	Leukotrienes (LTC4, D4, B4)	• TNF-α
• Tryptase + chymase	β-glucosaminidase	• Slow-reacting substance of anaphylaxis (SRSA)	
• Neutrophil + eosinophilic chemotactic factors			

MAST CELL GROWTH FACTOR

- Also known as stem-cell growth factor; melanocyte growth factor, Steel factor
- Receptor encoded by c-*kit* protooncogene, mutated in piebaldism.
- Increased in mastocytosis (urticaria pigmentosum).
- c-*kit* protooncogene encodes tyrosine kinase receptor, which stem/mast cell growth factor binds
- Mutations in c-*kit* constitutively activate mast cell proliferation.

EFFECTS OF PROSTAGLANDIN D2

- Vasodilation
- Neutrophil chemotaxis
- Platelet inhibition
- Bronchoconstriction
- Eosinophil activation
- Mediates flushing secondary to niacin

TABLE 1–15
COMPOSITION OF SEBUM

Content	Sebum	Epidermal Lipids[a]
Glycerides	57.5%	65%
Wax esters	26%	0%
Squalene	12%	0%
Cholesterol esters	3%	15%
Cholesterol	1.5%	20%

[a] Free fatty acids on skin, not in glands.

T-CELL MARKERS

Pan T-cell: "prime numbers": CD 2, 3, 5, 7

TABLE 1–16
T-HELPER CELL STORY

Th1	Th2
Cell-mediated	Humoral-mediated
IL-2	IL-4
IL-12[a]	IL-5
IFN-γ	IL-10
TNF-β (lymphotoxin)	IL-13
TNF-α	
Psoriasis, rheumatoid arthritis	Atopic dermatitis
Mycosis fungoides (CTCL)	Sézary syndrome
Tuberculoid leprosy	Lepromatous leprosy
Tuberculosis (lupus vulgaris)	Miliary tuberculosis
Leishmania, granulomas	Diffuse leishmaniasis
Contact dermatitis (subsequent)	Contact dermatitis (elicitation)
Behçet syndrome (pathergy test)	Hypereosinophilia syndrome
Alopecia areata, vitiligo	

[a] IL-12 knockout mouse: increased susceptibility to mycobacterial infections.

UVB-INDUCED DNA MUTATIONS

1. Cyclobutane pyrimidine dimers
2. 6–4 Pyrimidine/pyrimidone dimers
3. Thymidine dimers [most common base-pair change: cytosine (C) → thymine (T)]

CHAPTER

2

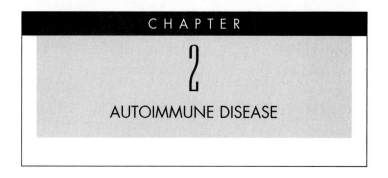

AUTOIMMUNE DISEASE

ANTIPHOSPHOLIPID ANTIBODIES

1. Also known as:
    - Anticardiolipin antibodies = identify by ELISA or radioimmunoassay
    - Lupus anticoagulant = inhibits a phospholipid detected by APTT, kaolin clotting time (KCT), Russell viper venom time (dRVVT)
    - Biological false-positive serologic test for syphilis (VDRL)
2. Clinical features:
    - Livedo reticularis and thrombotic events (i.e., Sneddon syndrome)
    - Recurrent spontaneous abortions
    - Associated with SLE, ovarian cancer

TABLE 2–1
AUTOANTIBODIES

Antibodies to	Antigen	Fluorescence Pattern	Disease
dsDNA = nDNA[b]	Native DNA	**Peripheral/rim** (specific for)	SLE with renal disease[a]
			Low complement levels
ssDNA		Homogenous	Linear morphea
ENAs:	Extractable nuclear Ags	ALL Particulate = speckle	
Sm		**Speckled** (specific for)	SLE (specific), CNS, nephritis
U_1RNP	(small RNA)		MCTD, neonatal LE (no heart block)
Ro/La		Fine speckled	SCLE, neonatal, Sjögren syndrome, photosensitivity, lymphopenia, Rowell syndrome = LE plus erythema multiforme
Scl-70	DNA topoisomerase I		PSS (low renal risk)
Histone		**Homogenous** (specific for)	Drug-induced lupus
Nucleolar	RNA	**Nucleolar** (specific for)	PSS
Centromere	Kinetochore (mitochondria)	**Centromere** (specific for)	CREST
Antiphospholipid	Phospholipid		Thrombotic disease
Jo-1	Histidyl-tRNA synthetase	"Mechanic's hands" =	DM/PM, pulmonary fibrosis, neoplasm
Mi-2	Nuclear helicase	Gottron's sign	Classic DM, best prognosis, Shawl sign
SRP	Signal-recognition particle		PM, cardiac, myalgias, acute, poor prognosis
MAS	Cytoplasmic RNA		PM, alcoholic rhabdomyolysis
Ku			Overlap CTD + dermatomyositis

c-ANCA	Proteinase-3	Cytoplasmic	Wegener's granulomatosis
p-ANCA	Myeloperoxidase, elastase, cathepsin G, lactoferrin, lysozyme, catalase	Perinuclear	Churg-Strauss (occ. PAN), drug-induced, IBD, cystic fibrosis
Other:			
rRNP			CNS involvement
RA-33			Erosive arthritis
RPP	Ribosomal P protein		Psychosis
zDNA	Left-handed double helix		Some SLE patients

[a] Order of improvement in LE with treatment: (1) nephritis, (2) C-reactive protein, (3) ESR, (4) autoantibody.

[b] *Crithida lucilae* = substrate for dsDNA in lab; HEP-2 cells = human laryngeal carcinoma cells act as substrate for ANA in lab.

TABLE 2–2
ANA PATTERNS

Fluorescence	Specific for	Antigen
Peripheral/rim	SLE	dsDNA
Homogenous	Drug-induced SLE	Histone
Nucleolar	Scleroderma	Nucleolar
Centromere	CREST	Kinetochore
Speckled	MCTD	U_1RNP

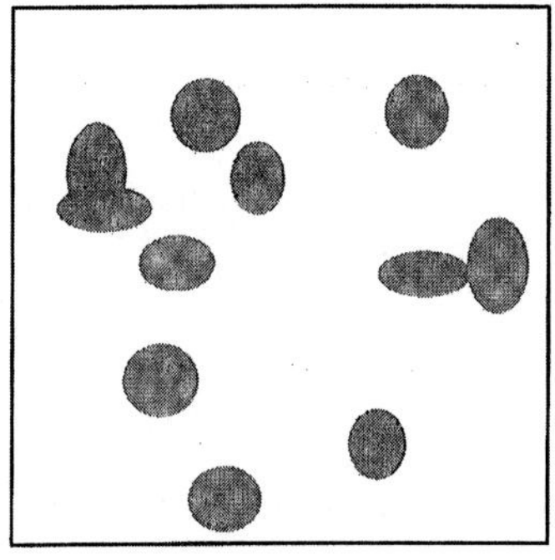

Homogenous pattern

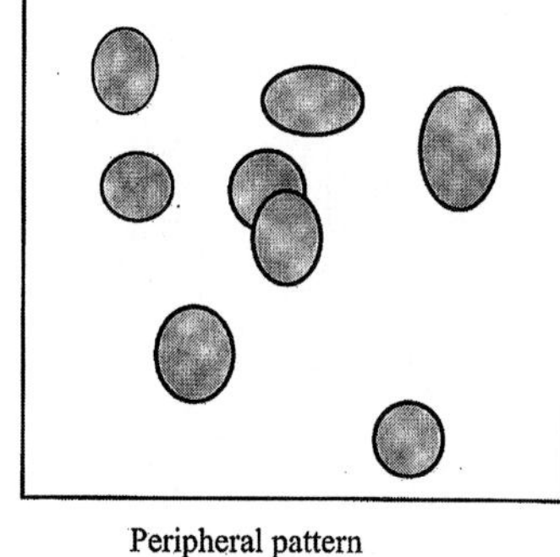

Peripheral pattern

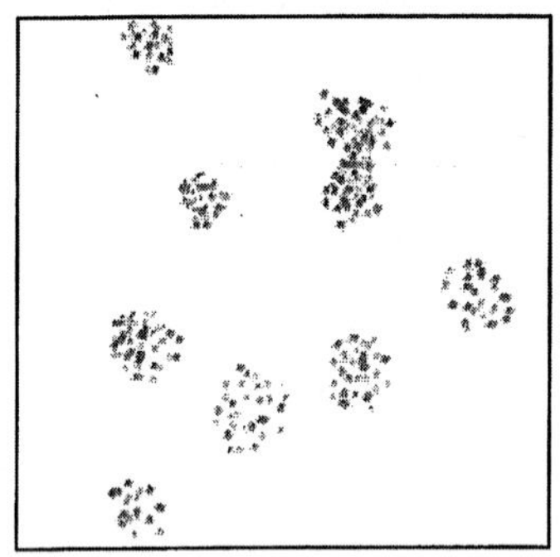

Speckled pattern

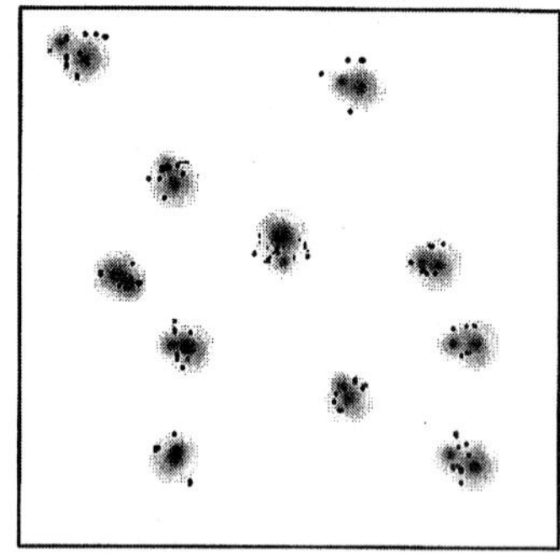

Nucleolar pattern

FIGURE 2–1
ANA immunofluorescence patterns.

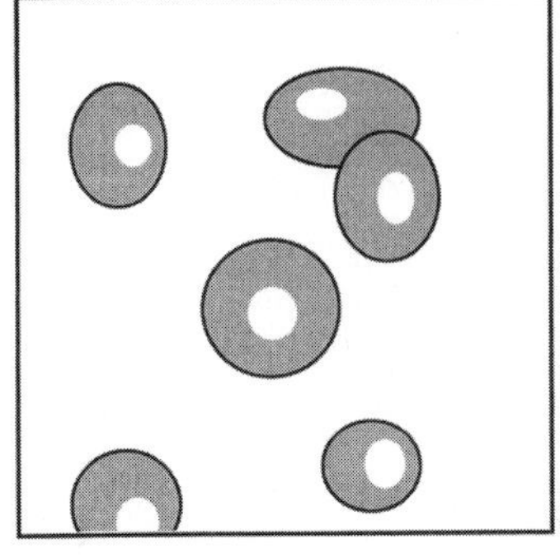

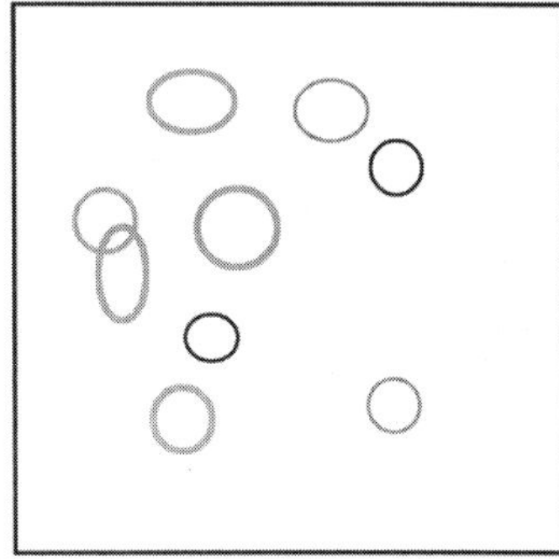

c-ANCA p-ANCA

FIGURE 2–2
ANCA immunofluorescence patterns.

CHURG-STRAUSS SYNDROME

American College of Rheumatology (ACR) criteria = +4/6

1. Asthma
2. Eosinophilia >10%
3. Neuropathy
4. Pulmonary infiltrate
5. Sinus abnormality
6. Extravascular eosinophils on biopsy (two-thirds with nodule on extremities or head)

- Most frequent cause of death: myocarditis resulting in CHF
- Drug-induced: zafirlukast, azithromycin, free-base cocaine, hepatitis B vaccination

TABLE 2–3
CRYOGLOBULINEMIA: CLASSIFICATION OF CRYOGLOBULINS

Type	Immunoglobulin Type	Immune Complex	Clinical	Associated Diseases
1	Monoclonal IgG or IgM	None	Purpura of the distal extremities, NO LCV	Lymphoproliferative: leukemia, lymphoma, myeloma, macroglobulinemia
2	Monoclonal/polyclonal	IgM-IgG	Palpable purpura (LCV)	Lymphoproliferative: leukemia, lymphoma, myeloma, macroglobulinemia; rheumatoid arthritis, hepatitis C (80%), Sjögren syndrome
3 (mixed)	Polyclonal/polyclonal	IgM-IgG	Palpable purpura (LCV)	Autoimmune: RA, SLE, Sjögren syndrome, Hepatitis B and C, mononucleosis (EBV), CMV, biliary cirrhosis

BROW–MNEMONIC FOR GLUTEN POSITIVE FOODS

B = barley
R = rye
O = oats
W = wheat

Gluten-free:
- Rice
- Potato

TABLE 2–4
CRITERIA FOR LUPUS ERYTHEMATOSUS

Skin	Systemic	Serologies	Inflammation
Photosensitivity	Renal	(+) ANA	Arthritis
Malar	Neurologic	Other antibodies	Serositis
Discoid	Heme		
Oral ulcers			

TABLE 2–5
(SYSTEMIC LUPUS DIAGNOSTIC CRITERIA)[a]

M	Malar rash
D	Discoid lesions
S	Serositis
O	Oral ulcers
A	ANA positivity
P	Photosensitivity
B	Blood/heme (anemia, WBC)
R	Renal
A	Arthritis
I	Immunologic (other autoantibodies)
N	Neurologic

[a] Mnemonic for types of lesions.

TABLE 2–6
LUPUS-BAND TEST (DIRECT IMMUNOFLUORESCENCE TEST)

	SLE	SCLE	DLE
Lesional	90%	50%	80%
Nonlesional	70%	30%	10%
ANA+	>90%	60%	35%

TABLE 2–7
DRUG-INDUCED LUPUS ERYTHEMATOSUS (LE)[a]

INE	IDE	Other
Chlorpromazine	Isoniazid	Methyldopa
Hydralazine	Procainamide	Diethylstilbestrol (DES)
Penicillamine	Sulfonamide	Hydroxyurea
Quinidine	Aminoglutethimide	Tegafur
Phenytoin	Leuprolide	
Minocycline		

[a] Antihistone-positive *except* penicillamine, which is anti-dsDNA-positive.

TABLE 2–8
DRUG-INDUCED SYSTEMIC LUPUS ERYTHEMATOSUS (SCLE)

Thiazides	Griseofulvin	ACE inhibitors (captopril)
Aldactone	Sulfonylureas	
Piroxicam	Procainamide	
Naproxen	Oxyprenolol	Calcium channel blockers
Penicillamine	Phenothiazine	(diltiazem, verapamil, nifedipine)
Gold	Beta blockers	

LUPUS (SCLE) ASSOCIATIONS

- Photosensitivity
- +ANA (80%)
- Arthritis (75%)
- Alopecia (50%)
- Hard palate lesions (40%)
- Leukopenia (20%)
- HLA-DR3

TABLE 2–9
POLYARTERITIS NODOSA: CUTANEOUS VS. SYSTEMIC

	Systemic	Cutaneous
Blood pressure	↑	Normal
M:F ratio	2:1	1:1
WBC	↑	Normal to moderate
Eosinophils	↑	Increase
Proteinuria	↑	Normal
Visceral	yes	Normal
involvement	fatal in 2 years with no treatment	None
Prognosis		Chronic, relapsing, benign 10% progress to systemic

RHO (ρ) ANTIBODY ASSOCIATED WITH:

- SCLE/SLE (30%)
- Sjögren syndrome (45%)
- Neonatal lupus
- Homozygous C_2 and C_4 deficiency
- Late-onset LE
- Mothers of infants with neonatal LE (90%)
- Rowell syndrome (lupus plus erythema multiforme) = anti-la
- ANA (–) lupus = 60% have + Rho
- HLA-DR3
- Photosensitivity
- Malar rash
- Drug induced SCLE (thiazides) (70%)
- Normal individuals (0–5%)

RHO (ρ) ANTIBODY PLUS NEONATAL LUPUS

- 1% of Ro+ pregnant mothers → baby with neonatal lupus.
- 10% of neonatal lupus patients → congenital heart block.
- If first pregnancy = neonatal lupus, 25% of second pregnancy = neonatal lupus.

SCLERODERMA (PSS)

- Fibrous thickening of skin + fibrosis/vascular abnormalities of internal organs.
- Raynaud phenomenon is the first manifestation in >50% patients.
- Initially, skin is erythematous and swollen; commonly misdiagnosed as carpal tunnel syndrome.
- Face becomes expressionless, hands become claw-like (sclerodactyly), lips are radially furrowed.
- Neck sign: ridging and tightening of neck on extension in >90% of patients.
- Round finger pad sign: pad loses pulp.
- Pterygium inversum unguis: distal nail plate becomes adherent to nail bed via hyponychium.
- Prominent, tortuous nail fold capillaries; if bleeding, 90% specific for PSS.
- Hands more severely affected than feet.
- Diffuse calcification and diffuse hyperpigmentation.
- Hypopigmentation → perifollicular hyperpigmentation.
- Decreased sweat gland activity.
- Pulmonary fibrosis: honeycomb change in lungs.
- Esophageal and intestinal atonia.
- Cardiac conduction defects.
- Death occurs from renal and cardiac changes (use captopril to treat acute episode).

SHAWL SIGN

V-neck photosensitivity in dermatomyositis patients.

STILL'S DISEASE (JUVENILE RHEUMATOID ARTHRITIS)

Rash occurs in the afternoon; rapidly resolves; looks like gyrate erythema or tinea corporis.

CHAPTER

3

INFLAMMATORY DERMATOSES

TABLE 3–1
DIFFERENTIAL DIAGNOSIS OF ACRAL PURPURA

Infectious	Collagen Vascular	Embolic
Subacute bacterial endocarditis	Leukocytoclastic vasculitis	Left atrial myxoma
Rocky Mountain spotted fever	Polyarteritis nodosa	Cholesterol emboli
Gonococcemia	Lupus erythematosus	Traumatic aneurysm
Sepsis	Wegener's granulomatosis	
Hepatitis C and cryoglobulinemia		
Parvovirus B19		
Vasoocclusive	**Dysproteinemic**	
Atherosclerosis	Cryoglobulinemia	
Antiphospholipid antibody syndrome	Cryofibrinogenemia	
Sneddon syndrome (idiopathic livedo reticularis with stroke and hypertension)	Hyperglobulinemic purpura	

AIRBORNE/RAGWEED DERMATITIS

1. Plant family Compositae
2. Antigen: Sesquiterpene lactone
3. Plants
   - Eucerin and ultravate
   - Ragweed
   - Chrysanthemum (pyrethrin): used in Elimite®
   - Liverwort (*Frullenia*): not Compositae, but contains sesquiterpene lactone
   - Parthenium (feverfew): scourge of India
   - Lettuce
   - Sage
   - Artichoke
   - Turpentine
   - Arnica
   - Chamomile
   - Chicory
   - Marigold
   - Hempweed
   - Laurel oil
   - Sunflower
   - Tansy
   - Tulip tree
   - Yarrow
   - Philodendron
   - English ivy
   - Prairie crocus
   - Grevillea
   - Dieffenbachia
   - Peruvian lily
4. Patch test: uses sesquiterpene lactone mix

ALLYL DISULFIDE

Contact allergen also found in:

- Garlic
- Chives
- Leeks
- Onions

AMMONIUM PERSULFATE

- Bleaching (hair)
- Contact urticaria

BALSAM OF PERU

Cosmetic fragrance; has cinnamon and vanilla odor

1. Antigen: Cinnamein (oil) contains cinnamic alcohol, cinnamic aldehyde, methyl cinnamate, benzyl cinnamate, vanillin, eugenol, and benzoic acid
2. Cross reacts with:
   - Chocolate
   - Tincture of benzoin
   - Cough syrup
   - Cinnamon oil
   - Clove oil
   - Citrus peel

BEHÇET SYNDROME

Th1 disease involving:

- Oral/genital aphthae, uveitis, synovitis, vasculitis, thromboses, meningo-encephalitis, HLA-B51.
- Eye involvement: posterior uveitis > conjunctivitis > corneal ulceration > papilledema > arteritis.

- MAGIC syndrome = Behçet and relapsing polychondritis.
- Cardiac manifestations associated with concurrent deficiency of protein S.

BLEPHARITIS

Caused by:

- Seborrheic dermatitis
- Staphylococcal
- Molluscum contagiosum
- Rosacea
- Mixed species
- Pediculosis

TABLE 3–2
DEFICIENCY OF C1 ESTERASE INHIBITOR: NO URTICARIA, ONLY ASYMMETRICAL SWELLING

	C1	C4	C2	C3	C1-INH	C1q	CH50	Associations
Hereditary (Quincke's disease)	nl	↓	↓	nl	↓ (protein nl)	↓	nl/↓	Spares periorbital area
Hereditary (variant, 15%)	nl	↓	↓	nl	nl (abnormal protein)	↓	nl/↓	
Acquired (Caldwell's)	↓	↓	↓	nl	↓/nl		↓	Type 1: B-cell lymphoma Type 2: idiopathic

[a] Chronic urticaria is associated with antibody against α chain of F_cERI.
[b] Treat: acute episodes (2–4 days) with fresh frozen plasma, chronic with dantrolene sodium (Danazol®) (does not work for type 2 acquired).
[c] Check C1 levels to differentiate between acquired and hereditary forms.

CHEMICALS THAT GO THROUGH CONVENTIONAL (LATEX) GLOVES

- Nickel
- Cobalt
- Formaldehyde
- Glutaraldehyde
- Acrylates
- Epoxy resins
- Thioglycolate

CHROMIUM

Contact allergen in cement; also used leather tanning, causing "blackjack" felt dermatitis. Cross-reacts with nickel.

COBALT

Present in injections of vitamin B_{12}. When given to patients with pernicious anemia, causes increased sensitivity. Coreacts with nickel.

COLOPHONY

Resinous substance from tree sap used as an adhesive; causes contact dermatitis. Also found in

- Band-Aids
- Turpentine
- Lacquers
- Varnishes
- Rosin
- Abeitic acid (mascara)
- Chewing gum (perioral dermatitis)
- Newspapers (hand dermatitis)

COSMETICS PRESERVATIVES

The following may cause contact dermatitis:

- Imidazolidinyl urea: formaldehyde releaser, second most common allergen.
- Quaternium-15: formaldehyde releaser (most common cause of preservative-induced dermatitis).
- Quaternium-18-bentonite = ivy block.
- Polyquaternium-10 = active ingredient in hair conditioners.
- Parabens: most often used topical preservative, least frequent allergen. *not* a formaldehyde releaser. Allergen in amide anesthetics and Accutane.
- EUXYL K 400 = methyl dibromoglutaronitrile; found in facial tissues and toilet paper.
- Kathon CG = methylchloroisothiazolinone; found in Eucerine®, Ultravate®, shampoos and conditioners.
- Formaldehyde releasers in wrinkle-free clothing.

CUTTING OILS

- Insoluble cutting oils cause folliculitis.
- Soluble cutting oils cause allergic contact dermatitis.

ALLERGENS IN DENTISTRY

Common contact allergens:

- Glutaraldehyde
- Rubber/latex
- Resins (acrylates)

DIFFERENTIAL DIAGNOSIS OF DIAPER DERMATITIS

- Irritant/allergic
- Psoriasis
- Seborrheic dermatitis
- Langerhans cell histiocytosis (histiocytosis X)
- Granuloma gluteale infantum
- Acrodermatitis enteropathica
- Chronic bullous disease of childhood
- Candidal infection
- Jacquet dermatitis (pseudoverrucous papules)

ETHYLENEDIAMINE

Contact allergen present in the following:

- Aminophylline (theophylline and ethylenediamine)
- Atarax
- Nystatin cream
- Meclizine

EUXYL K 400 (METHYLDIBROMOGLUTARONITRILE)

- Cosmetic preservative; may cause contact dermatitis.
- Found in facial tissues and toilet paper (in Europe).

TABLE 3–3
FIGURATE ERYTHEMAS

Disease	Characteristics
Erythema annulare centrifugum	Slow-moving, seen on trunk, idiopathic
Erythema gyratum repens	Rapidly moving, concentric "wood grain," cancer marker
Erythema (chronicum) migrans	Originating from tick bite
Erythema marginatum	Rapidly spreading, RF-specific, fleeting; check ASO titer
Familial annular erythema	Autosomal dominant; rare
Annular erythema of infancy	Rule out lupus

FLORISTS

Common contact allergens

- Chrysanthemum: sesquiterpene lactone
- Tuliposide A: *Alstromeria*
- Tulipaline A = Peruvian lily, Philodendron, English ivy, Prairie crocus, *Grevillea*, *Parthenium*
- Tulip and daffodils: oxalate (bulb-sorter's disease)

GLUTARALDEHYDE

- Disinfectant and preservative used as cold-sterilizing agent in medicine and dentistry
- Contact allergen found in Cidex®

HAIR

Common contact allergens

- Permanent waving solutions: Glyceryl monothioglycolate
- Black hair dye: paraphenylenediamine (PPD); also in color developers and scuba gear
- Bleach contains ammonium persulfate; may cause contact urticaria or anaphylaxis
- Depilatories: thioglycolates dissolve disulfide bonds = 15% hair, 2% skin
- Shampoo surfactant contains cocamidopropyl betaine
- Conditioner = polyquaternium-10

HALOGENODERMAS

- Iodides (more likely to ulcerate), fluorides = on face
- Bromides = on leg
- Pseudoepitheliomatous hyperplasia, suppurative granulomas, verrucous lesions with peripheral pustules

TABLE 3–4
IRRITANT DERMATITIS

Milky Sap	Oxalate Crystals	Capsaicin	Caterpillars
Poinsettia	Tulips Daffodils (bulb sorter's disease)	Hot peppers	Puss (fur ball) Io (green with red stripe)

DIFFERENTIAL DIAGNOSIS OF ITCHY RED BUMPS

- Scabies
- Atopic dermatitis
- Grover's disease
- Dermatographism/physical urticaria

- Insect bite = papular urticaria
- Dermatitis herpetiformis
- Contact dermatitis
- Pityriasis lichenoides et varioliformis acuta (PLEVA)
- Papular eruption of black men
- Prurigo simplex subacuta
- Itchy red bump disease

KAWASAKI DISEASE

Treat with IVIG and ASA (also dipyrimadole)

- 5 days of high fever
- Bilateral conjunctival injection
- Strawberry tongue, fissures
- Cervical lymphadenopathy
- Polymorphous exanthem (morbilliform)
- Red lips
- Palmar/sole erythema and edema
- Coronary aneurysm (10% of patients; 70% with ECG changes)
- Leading cause of death = myocardial infarction

VARIANTS OF KERATOSIS PILARIS

1. Ulerythema oophorogenes: lateral eyebrows
2. Keratosis pilaris atrophicans facei: atrophic scarring
3. Atrophodermia vermiculata: "worm-eaten honeycomb" atrophy on face
4. Keratosis pilaris rubra
5. Keratosis pilaris
6. Erythromelanosis follicularis facei et colli: hyperpigmented lateral cheeks
7. Keratosis follicularis spinulosa decalvans: scalp with scarring alopecia (X-linked recessive)

TABLE 3–5
KIMURA DISEASE VS. ANGIOLYMPHOID HYPERPLASIA WITH EOSINOPHILIA

Kimura Disease	Angiolymphoid Hyperplasia with Eosinophilia
Negative HHV8	Positive HHV8
Lymphadenopathy present	No lymphadenopathy
Deep, nontender	Red, superficial, tender
Renal involvement	No renal changes

LANOLIN

Lanolin alcohol (e.g., wool alcohol, wool fat, wool grease, wool wax) is a contact allergen in prescription creams and cosmetics.

LATEX

- Cross-reacts with ABC: avocado, banana, chestnut—also kiwi, passion fruit, peach, mango, pineapple, fig, cantaloupe, apple, papaya, ethylene-ripened fruits.

- Risk factors: spina bifida, female gender, repeated urinary catheterization, repeated fecal impaction, other congenital anomalies.
- Increased IgE → most effective predictor of anaphylaxis to latex.
- PBC gloves, polymethane condoms, and polychloroprene do not contain latex.

1. Type 1 hypersensitivity: IgE-mediated; caused by small latex particles, worse on broken skin/genitalia; RAST test.
2. Type 4 hypersensitivity: cell-mediated type caused by accelerators, antioxidants, emulsifiers; patch testing elicits reaction.

TABLE 3–6
LEUKOCYTOCLASTIC VASCULITIS (IMMUNOLOGIC)

Immune Complex	Direct Antibody	ANCA	Cell-Mediated	Idiopathic
Cryoglobulins	Goodpasture	Wegener	Allograft	Giant-cell arteritis
Henoch-Schönlein	Kawasaki	Churg-Strauss		Takayasu
Lupus		PAN		
Rheumatoid arthritis		Microscopic polyangiitis		
Behçet disease				
Paraneoplastic				
Serum sickness				

DIFFERENTIAL DIAGNOSIS OF LEUKOCYTOCLASTIC VASCULITIS (INFECTIOUS—EMBOLIC)

- Gonococcemia
- SBE
- Spirochete
- Viral (HSV)
- Meningococcemia
- Rickettsial
- Mucor (fungal)
- Mycobacterial

NAIL POLISH

Common contact allergens:

- Toluenesulfonamide/formaldehyde resin
- Methacrylate (artificial nails)
- Resorcinol (yellow color)

NICKEL

Most common metal allergen: dimethylglyoxime test

PABA CROSS-REACTIONS: (MNEMONIC "PABA PLUS PASTE")

- **PABA**
- **P**PD

- **A**zo dyes
- **S**ulfonamides/sullfonylureas
- **T**hiazides
- **E**ster anesthetics: benzocaine, cocaine, procaine, tetracaine, dibucaine

PATHERGY

Th1 disease, associated with

- Sweet disease
- Pyoderma gangrenosum
- Bowel bypass
- Behçet disease

DIFFERENTIAL DIAGNOSIS OF PERFORATING DERMATOSES

- Perforating folliculitis
- Perforating collagenosis (reactive)
- Perforating disorder of renal failure
- Perforating GA
- Perforating PXE (perforating calcific elastosis)
- Kyrle disease
- EPS

TABLE 3–7
PHOTOTOXIC VS. PHOTOALLERGIC

Characteristics	Phototoxic	Photoallergic
Appearance	Sunburn	Eczematous
Action spectrum	UVA + UVB	UVA
Reaction	Direct cell damage	DTH
Reaction to first exposure	Yes	No
Timing	Rapid	Delayed
Antigen concentration	High	Low
Pathology	Basal degeneration	Acute spongiotic dermatitis

PHYTOPHOTODERMATITIS

1. Phototoxic with UVA
2. Plant family: Ubelliferae (U) or Rutaceae (R)

TABLE 3–8
COMMON CAUSES OF PHYTOPHOTODERMATITIS

Fruits/Vegetables	Perfumes[a]
Lemon/lime (R)	Oil of bergamot
Parlsey (U)	5-Methoxypsoralen
Celery (celery root) (U)	
Parsnips	
Carrot greens (U)[b]	
Orange (R)	
Mango (R)	
Coriander (U)	
Grapefruit	

[a] Berloque (dermatitis) = lavaliere sign = hanging-drop sign.
[b] Citrus items are in the family Rutacea, greens are in the family Umbelliferae.

TYPES OF PIGMENTED PURPURA

1. Majocchi = purpura annularis telangiectoides
2. Schaumberg = progressive pigmentary dermatosis (cayenne pepper)
3. Gougerot and Blum = pigmented purpuric lichenoid dermatitis
4. Doucas and Kapetanakis = eczematoid-like purpura
5. Lichen aureus = localized variant; "gold" color

POISON IVY/RHUS

1. Plant family: Anacardiaceae
   - Plant group Toxicodendron includes poison ivy, oak, sumac
2. Antigen: Pentadecylcatechol from oleoresin (dry resin) or urushiol (milky secretion)
3. Cross-reacting substances:

CALAMARI with **GIN**ger and **PEPPER**	**OTHER STUFF**
CAshew nut oil + shells	**P**epeo tree (Venezuela)
LAcquer tree of Japan	**El** litre tree (Chile)
Mango **R**ind (not juice)	**R**engas tree (black varnish tree, Malaya)
Indian marking tree	
GINgko tree (leaf pulp – not in supplement	
PEP (Brazilian pepper)	

JOINT MANIFESTATIONS OF PSORIASIS (HLA B27)

1. Asymmetrical DIP with positive nail changes
2. Arthritis mutilans with osteolysis

3. Symmetrical polyarthritis like RA
4. Oligoarthritis (most common—70%)
5. Ankylosing spondylitis

DIFFERENTIAL DIAGNOSIS OF STELLATE PURPURA

Meningococcemia
Cryoglobulins
Protein C deficiency
Systemic polyarteritis nodosa
Calcium deposition in vessels
Cholesterol emboli/atheromas: cold sensation + dull ache

PYODERMA GANGRENOSUM ASSOCIATED WITH

Arthritis (rheumatoid)
Inflammatory bowel disease
Leukemia (AML)
IgA paraproteinemia
Hypogammaglobulinemia
Sarcoid
Chronic active hepatitis
Collagen vascular disease
Multiple myeloma

TABLE 3–9
RUBBER MIXES

Rubber Mix	Type	Clinical
Thiuram	Accelerator	Active ingredient in Antabuse, primary cause of glove dermatitis
Mercaptobenzothiazole	Accelerator	Most common cause of shoe dermatitis (spares instep + webspaces)
P-Phenylenediamine (PPD)	Oxidizer	Cross-reacts with PPD in hair dyes, color developers, and scuba gear
Carba	Accelerator	Cross reacts with thiuram
Zinc dibenzylthiocarbamate		Allergenic when bleached = underwear elastic-band dermatitis
Hydroquinone	Oxidizer	
Latex		Cross reacts with ABC: avocado, banana, chestnut

TYPES OF SARCOID

- Lupus pernio: nasal alae, perioral area, ears, digits; +/– violaceous edematous plaque; 75% severe lung disease; 40% severe bone involvement.
- Periorbital papules in African Americans may be sarcoid.

TABLE 3–10
SARCOIDOSIS SYNDROME—GRANULOMATOUS INFECTION

Lofgren's Triad[b]	Heerfordt's Triad (Uveoparotid Fever)[a]	Darier-Roussy Sarcoid	Mikulicz Syndrome
Hilar adenopathy Erythema nodosum (good prognosis) Polyarthritis[c]	Uveitis Parotiditis Facial (seventh) nerve palsy	Subcutaneous nodules on trunk and extremities	Involvement of bilateral parotid, submandibular, sublingual, and lacrimal glands

[a] 90% of visceral involvement is lung and intrathoracic lymph nodes; most common cause of death = cor pulmonale.
[b] Eye finding: "mutton fat" precipitates in anterior chamber.
[c] Osseous granulomas cause sausage digits.
[d] Systemic: check ACE levels or Kveim skin test; gallium scan may show panda or lambda signs.
[e] Treatment: (1) steroids, (2) antimalarials, (3) MTX, (4) allopurinol, (5) thalidomide.

TIXOCORTOL PIVALATE

Contact allergen in topical steroids

THIMEROSAL

Preservative that can cause contact dermatitis. Found in the following:

- Vaccines (children can be sensitized to it)
- Contact lens solution
- Eye shadow
- Gammaglobulin

TOOTHPASTE

Contains contact allergen cinnamic aldehyde.

VITAMIN E

α-Tocopherol (synthetic vitamin E) is incorporated into deodorants and cosmetics and may cause contact allergic reactions.

CHAPTER 4

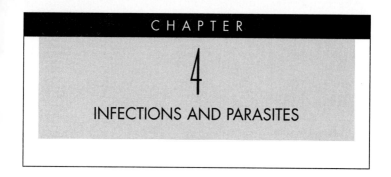

INFECTIONS AND PARASITES

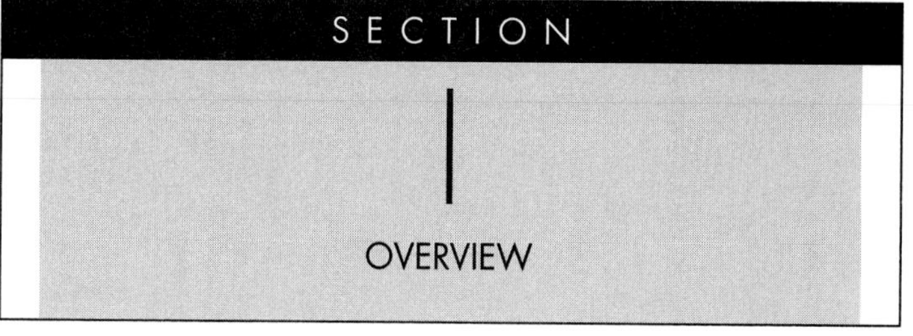

TABLE 4–1
BARTONELLA DISEASES: GRAM-NEGATIVE RODS

Genus/ Species	Cat Sctatch	Bacillary Angiomatosis	Trench Fever	Oroya Fever or Verruca Peruana (Bartonellosis)	Endocarditis	Peliosis Hepatis	Reservoir + Vector
B. henselae	+	+			+	+	Cat flea
B. quintana		(occasional +)	+		+		Body louse
B. bacilliformis				+			Sandfly
B. elizabethae					+		
B. clarridgeiae	+						Cat
B. miscellanei							
Other	Treatment: Erythromycin or doxycycline			Mortality when coinfected with *Salmonella*			

[a]The most common complication of cat-scratch fever is central nervous system involvement.

TABLE 4–2
BITES

Animal/ Disease	Family or Genus/Species	Region	Clinical Manifestations	Markings or Toxic Effect	Treatment
Brown recluse[a]	*Loxosceles reclusa*	South, Midwest, South America	Painful bite, hemorrhagic blister, necrosis, red-white-blue; rarely systemic	Inverted "violin" on thorax Sphingomyelinase D [[AU 4]]= phospholipase = hemolysis	First: RICE (rest, ice, compression, elevation) Second: Dapsone Third: Excision
Black widow[a]	*Lactrodactus mactans*	USA (48 states)	Painless sting, muscle paralysis, surgical abdomen, respiratory paralysis	Abdomen: red hourglass patch Have neurotoxins	Symptomatic
Tarantula	Theraphosidae		Hairs → urticaria		
Hymenopterae (bees, wasps)		USA (48 states)	Severe bites		Apply ASA + papain
Scorpion		Southwest	Circular bites, head & neck	Neurotoxin + hemolysis	
Saddleback caterpillar	*Sibine stimulea*		Linear; hairs → irritation Histamine = itching	"Saddlebag" markings on green caterpillar	
Puss caterpillar	*Megalopyge opercularis*		Pain = stinging; hemolysis	Fur-ball–like rabbit's foot	

TABLE 4–2
BITES (*Continued*)

Animal/ Disease	Family or Genus/Species	Region	Clinical Manifestations	Markings or Toxic Effect	Treatment
Io caterpillar	*Automeris io*		Pain = stinging; hemolysis	Colorful green/yellow with red and white stripe	
Centipede			Poisonous bite		
Blister beetle			Blistering	Brown color, source of cantharidin	
Dog/cat mites	*Cheyletiella*		"Walking dandruff"	Scabies with long legs	
Grain mite	*Pyemotes ventricosus*		Many bites in areas of constricted clothing		
Fowl mite	*Dermanyssus gallinae/avium*				
Fire ant	*Solenopsis saevissima*		Very painful, many bites lead to sterile pustules; cross-reacts with bee stings	Solenopsin D toxin: hemolysis + histamine	
Sand flea	*Tunga penetrans*	Chigoe flea	Black dot on sole	No wings, long legs	

Haverhill rat bite fever	*Streptobacillus moniliformis*	Haverhill, MA	Rash on joints, arthritis, fever		Penicillin, doxycycline, erythromycin
Rat bite fever (Sodoku)	*Spirillum minus*		Rash, fever		Penicillin, doxycycline
Dog bite infection, cat bite infection	*Capnocytophaga canimosus* *Pasteurella multocida*		Immunocompromised host = sepsis		Penicillin, doxycycline
Human bite infection	-*Eikenella corrodens*		Swelling, cellulitis, lymphadenopathy		Penicillin bactrim clindamycin
Poisonous snakes			Anaphylaxis, fever, serum sickness	Elliptical pupils, fangs	Compression, limb splint; identify venom
Tick	*Ixodes*		*Borrelia* lymphocytoma = blue nodule: earlobe (children), nipple, scrotum, nose (adults)		
Bats			Rabies Inhalation of bat feces → histoplasmosis		

[a] Lindane kills spiders.

BLASTOMYCOSIS (NORTH AMERICAN)

- Sporotrichoid spread, dog bites, beaver dams
- Treat with itraconazole (or amphotericin B, fluconazole)

TABLE 4–3
DIFFERENTIAL DIAGNOSIS OF "BLUEBERRY MUFFIN" LESIONS[a]

Dermal Erythropoiesis	Neoplastic-Infiltrative Diseases
Congenital infection	Neuroblastoma
• Rubella (deafness, glaucoma, cataracts most common, CHDs)	Congenital leukemia (chloroma)
• CMV (chorioretinitis, deafness, hepatosplenomegaly, mitral regurgitation)	Rhabdomyosarcoma
• Toxoplasmosis	Histiocytosis
• Varicella	
• AIDS	
• Parvovirus B19	
Hemolytic disease of the newborn	
• Rh incompatibility	
• Blood group incompatibility	
Hereditary spherocytosis	
Twin-twin transfusion syndrome	

[a] "Torch" mnemonic: ***T**oxoplasma*, **o**ther (syphilis), **r**ubella, **C**MV, **H**SV.

SPECIATION TESTS FOR *CANDIDA ALBICANS*

- Sucrose assimilation test
- Cornmeal Tween agar: enables *Candida* to form chlamydoconidia
- Germ tube test

CANDIDAL ONYCHOMYCOSIS

Affecting the fingernails, occurs most commonly in diabetics or people who handle sugar syrup or subject their hands to immersion (e.g., food handlers).

- weekly fluconazole treatment of choice

TABLE 4–4
THE "CHIGGER/CHIGOE" STORY

Chigger	Scrub typhus (tsutsugamushi fever)
Chigoe flea	Tungiasis (*Tunga penetrans*)
Chiclero ulcer	*Leishmania mexicana*

COCCIDIOIDOMYCOSIS

- Cutaneous: primary or disseminated from lung
- Primary pulmonary; 20% have cutaneous lesions
- Spontaneous recovery usually; fluconazole best treatment
- Poor prognosis and higher prevalence in males, Hispanics, Native Americans, Filipinos, infants and elderly, blood groups B or AB, and AIDS patients

TABLE 4–5
CORYNEBACTERIUM INFECTIONS

Disease	Species
Pitted keratolysis	*Micrococcus sedentarius*
Trichomycosis axillaris	*Corynebacterium tenius*
Erythrasma	*Corynebacterium minutissimum*
Shunt/tube infections	Groups J and K (also *Propionibacterium acnes*)

COXSACKIE A16 (AND A5): HAND-FOOT-MOUTH DISEASE; RNA VIRUS

- Follows dermatoglyphs (fingerprint lines)
- Herpangina: tonsillar/palate vesicles/erosions

CRYPTOCOCCUS

- Molluscum-like or abscesses
- "Pigeon droppings"
- Serology is false-positive if RA factor positive
- Capsule = blue with methylene + Alcian blue; = red with mucicarmine; India ink also used
- Treatment = amphotericin B followed by fluconazole

TABLE 4–6
DEMATIACEOUS FUNGI (PIGMENTED FUNGI THAT PRODUCE MELANIN)

DEEP			Superficial	Saprophytes
Eumycotic mycetoma	Chromomycosis	Phaeohyphomycosis	*Phaeoannellomyces wernekii*	*Alternaria*
Pseudallescheria	*Fonsecaea*	*Exophiala*	*Piedra hortae* (scalp)	Bipolaris
Madurella	*Phialophora*	*Wangiella*	*Trichosporum beigelii* (beard)	*Cladosporium*
Aspergillus	*Cladosporium*	*Alternaria*		*Curvularia*
Acremonium	*Rhinocladiella*			*Scopulariopsis* (nails)
PAMA	FRCP	EWA		ABCs

DEMODEX

- *Demodex folliculorum* occupies the hair follicles.
- *Demodex brevis* occupies the meibomian and sebaceous glands.

TABLE 4–7
DERMATOPHYTES AND FUNGI (COLONY/MICROCHARACTERISTICS)

Dermatophyte	Colony Appearance	Microscopic Appearance	Special Characteristics
Trichophyton rubrum	Cottony, dark red reverse	Birds on wire, pencil macroconidia	
T. tonsurans	Suede, red reverse	Balloons on wire; torpedo macroconidia	Thiamine
T. mentagrophytes	Woolly/silky/powdery (varied)	Grapes, spiral hyphae	Urease+, perforates hair KOH the underside of blister roof
T. schoenlenii	Glabrous cerebriform, unbaked pie dough	Favic chandeliers = "antlers"	
T. violaceum	Purple glabrous, cerebriform	Tortuous branching tangled hyphae	
T. verrucosum	Glabrous cerebriform, gray-white	Chains of conidia, antlers; rat-tail macrocon	Thiamine, inositol
T. concentricum	Glabrous cerebriform orange	Antler-like hyphae	Thiamine
T. megninii	Red reverse		Histidine
Epidermophyton floccosum	Velvety khaki, with pucker	Beaver tail macroconidia = snowshoes	
Microsporum canis	Hairy yellow (reverse) dog	Thick-walled; 6–16 septa	Grows on rice
M. gypseum	Granular sandy beach	Thin-walled, 4–6 septa	
M. cookei		Thick-walled gypseum	
M. nanum		Pig snout macroconidia	
M. ferrugineum	Glabrous cerebriform orange	Bamboo hyphae	

TABLE 4–7
DERMATOPHYTES AND FUNGI (COLONY/MICROCHARACTERISTICS) (*Continued*)

Dermatophyte	Colony Appearance	Microscopic Appearance	Special Characteristics
M. audouinii	Fluffy; salmon-peach reverse	Hyphae with rounded ends	
M. distortum		Distorted/curved like *M. canis*	
M. gallinae	Fast growth, red color diffuses	Round *Canis*, thin-walled	
M. vanbreuseghesimii		Long, 12 septa	
Sporothrix	Leather, chocolate color	37° = cigars, 25° = hyphae with daisies	
Blastomyces		37° = broad-based buds	
Paracoccidioides		37° = mariner's wheel (in macrophage)	
Histoplasma capsulatum		37° = Narrow bud + halo in histiocyte, 25° = hyphae with land mines	
Coccidioides		37° = spherule same-sized spores, 25° = boxcars alternating with blank conidia (spaces)	
Penicillium	Bright rainbow sherbet, red reverse	37° = cross-wall yeast, 25° = hand bones/broom	
Prototheca		Morula on H & E	Olecranon bursitis
Cryptococcus	Mucoid creamy white	Gelatinous capsule	Mucicarmine++
Aspergillus		Flowerlike: ball with chains of conidia	
Candida	Creamy white colony	Pseudohyphae	

Rhinosporidium		Very large spherule with different-sized spores	Mucicarmine++
Rhizopus (Mucor)	Salt + pepper, very quick growth (within 2 days)	Bud underneath stems (sporangium)	
Cladosporum		Broom (similar to penicillium)	
Rhinocladiella		Toilet brush or knotted club	
Phialophora		Vase of flowers	
Scopulariopsis		Chains of round conidia	
Fusarium		Sickle-shaped	
Geotrichium		Boxcars	
Nocardia	Chalky orange	Long thin-walled filaments	
Phaeoannellomyces wernekii (T. nigra)		Treat with keratolytics	

TABLE 4–8
DERMATOPHYTE (DIFFERENTIAL GROWTH CHARACTERISTICS)[a]

Dermatophyte	Pigment on PDA	Urease (medium turns red)	Hair Perforation	Polished Rice
T. rubrum	Cherry red	–	–	
T. mentagrophytes		+	+	
M. canis	Yellow[b]			⊕ Growth
M. audouinii	Salmon pink			–
(*Cryptococcus*)		+		

[a] Androgenic hormones inhibit growth of all fungi, especially androstenedione.
[b] "Dog eats rice looks yellow" = *M. canis*.

TABLE 4–9
DERMATOPHYTES WITH NUTRITIONAL REQUIREMENTS

Requirement	*Trichophyton* Species	Mnemonic
Thiamine	*Tonsurans*	
	Violaceum	
	Verrucosum	
Histidine	*Megninii*	
Niacin	*Equinum*	Horse needs niacin
Inositol	*Verrucosum*	Wart needs thiamine, inositol
Olive oil	*Malasezzia furfur*	

TABLE 4–10
DERMATOPHYTES WITH GLABROUS CEREBRIFORM COLONIES

Mnemonic	Species	Color
So	*T. schoenleinii*	Tan (unbaked pie dough)
Fine and	*M. ferrugineum*	Rust-orange
Very	*T. verrucosum*	Gray white or pale yellow
Very	*T. violaceum*	Violet
Cerebriform	*T. concentricum*	White to tan to brown (maturity)

TABLE 4–11
DIMORPHIC FUNGI: (GROW AS BOTH YEAST AND HYPHAE)

Deep Mycoses	Superficial Mycoses
Blastomycosis[a]	*Malassezia furfur*
Coccidioidomycosis	*Phaeoannellomyces wernekii*
Paracoccidioidomycosis[a]	*Trichosporon beigelii*
Histoplasmosis[a]	
Sporotrichosis[a]	
Penicillium marneffei[a]	

[a] Thermally dimorphic.

TABLE 4–12
ENDOTHRIX INFECTIONS[a,b]

Mnemonic	Species	Type
Say	***S**udanense*	African
Say	***S**choenleinii*	Common
Violet	***V**iolaceum*	Common
You're	***Y**aoundei*	African
Going	***G**ourvilii*	African
Right to	***R**ubrum*	Common
Town	***T**onsurans*	Common

[a] Mnemonic for all *Trichophyton* species; "Say say violet you're going right to town."
[b] Species that cannot infect hair: *E. floccosum* and *T. concentricum* (because of androgens).

TABLE 4–13
FLUORESCENT TINEA CAPITIS: PTERIDINE FLUORESCES[a]

Mnemonic	Dermatophyte	Ecto/Endothrix	Color
Gee	*M. gypseum*	Ecto	Yellow
All	*M. audouini*	Ecto	Yellow
Canis	*M. canis*	Ecto	Yellow
Do	*M. canis var distortum*	Ecto	Yellow
Fluoresce	*M. ferrugineum*	Ecto	Yellow
Sometimes	*T. schoenleinii*	ENDO (+ favus)	Blue-white

[a] Mnemonic: "Gee all canis do fluoresce sometimes."

Table 4–14
DIFFERENTIAL DIAGONOSIS OF FOLLICULITIS

Bacterial	Fungal/Yeast	Other
Gram ⊕ Gram (–) (treat with Accutane or appropriate antibiotics)	Dermatophyte *Pityrosporum*	Herpetic *Molluscum contagiosum*
Hot tub folliculitis: *Pseudomonas*	*Candida*	Syphilis Demodicidiosis

GRAM-POSITIVE RODS

These retain color because there is no lipid in their cell walls:

- *Nocardia*
- *Bacillus anthracis*
- *Clostridium difficile*
- *Actinomyces*
- *Erysipelothrix*
- *Corynebacterium*

HEPATITIS C

Associated with:

- Lichen planus (1–35%)
- PCT (40–60%)
- Cryoglobulinemia (40%) (mixed)
- Vasculitis
- Polyarteritis nodosa
- Necrolytic acral erythema
- Interferon α-treated patients may develop Psoriasis/psoriatic arthritis
- Pruritus (generalized)

HEPATITIS B

Associated with:

- Serum sickness (20–30%)
- Cryoglobulinemia (mixed)
- Dermatomyositis-like
- Gianotti-Crosti syndrome (Europe; associated with EBV in USA)
- Polyarteritis nodosa
- Lichen planus
- Pyoderma gangrenosum

DIFFERENTIAL DIAGNOSIS OF HERPESVIRUS

DNA virus → nucleus (i.e., intranuclear)

- Herpes simplex/varicella zoster (OKA vaccine)
- EBV/CMV = irregular large endothelial cells; both intranuclear and intracytoplasmic inclusions in CMV
- Simian herpesvirus (B virus)
- HHV-6 (roseola = sixth disease = exanthem subitum) = high fever, then rash
- HHV-8 (Kaposi sarcoma, Castleman disease, primary effusion lymphoma)

HISTOPLASMA CAPSULATUM

- 10% have erythema nodosum
- Most common pediatric manifestation: purpura
- Acquired via inhalation from feces of bats, starlings, chickens, and other bird species
- Amphotericin B best treatment

TABLE 4–15
CLINICAL MANIFESTATIONS OF VIRAL INFECTION

Virus	Features
HSV-1 + 2	Herpes labialis, eczema herpeticum, encephalitis, erythema multiforme; binds to FGF receptor
VZV	Chickenpox, shingles
EBV	Mononucleosis, hepatitis, oral hairy leukoplakia, Burkitt lymphoma, nasopharyngeal carcinoma, binds to CD21, hypocomplementemic urticarial vasculitis
CMV	Mono-like, hepatitis, pneumonia, retinitis, colitis, cutaneous ulcers
HHV-6	Exanthem subitum, roseola, sixth disease
HHV-7	Possible pityriasis rosea
HHV-8	Kaposi sarcoma, Castleman disease (paraneoplastic pemphigus, POEMS), Primary effusion lymphoma

TABLE 4–16
TYPES OF HUMAN PAPILLOMAVIRUS

HPV Type	Clinical Manifestations
HPV-1	Deep plantar (myrmecia)
HPV-2, 4	Common warts
HPV-3, 10, 27–29	Flat warts
HPV-5, 8	Epidermodysplasia verruciformis (25% malignant)/SCC
HPV-6, 11	Buschke-Lowenstein/laryngeal papillomas/ condyloma
HPV-7	Butcher's warts
HPV-13, 32	Focal epithelial hyperplasia (Heck disease) (Native Americans)
HPV-16, 34, 35	Periungual warts
HPV-16	Bowenoid papulosis/periungual SCC
HPV-16, 18, 31, 33, 51	Genital warts → cervical cancer
HPV-23b	Stucco keratoses
HPV-30	Laryngeal carcinoma
HPV-37	Keratoacanthomas
HPV-48	SCC in immunocompromised hosts
HPV-60	Plantar verrucous cysts
HPV-65	Pigmented warts

TABLE 4–17
TYPES OF IMPETIGO[a]

Entity	Associations/Cause
Impetigo herpetiformis	Pustular psoriasis in pregnancy (third trimester), hypocalcemia; treat with dapsone
Impetigo contagiosum	*Staphylococcus* (70%), *Streptococcus pyogenes*
Bullous impetigo	*S. aureus* group 2, phage 71

[a] See also Table 4–29, below, on diseases mediated by staph/strep.

TABLE 4–18
TREATMENT OF INFESTATIONS

Lice	1% permethrin, 0.5% malathion (twice to kill hatching progeny/nits; causes neuronal damage) Ivermectin (200 μg/kg) Petrolatum (for eyelash treatments) Can live 1 month without blood meal
Scabies	5% permethrin, ivermectin (200 mcg/kg), 6% sulfur (pregnancy, infants) Can live 2–3 days away from skin

TABLE 4–19
LEISHMANIASIS[a,b]

Location	Clinical	Sandfly Vectors	Subspecies
Old World Asia (wet, rural areas) Middle East (dry, urban areas) Africa, Mediterranean	Oriental/Delhi sore Baghdad boil All can cause recidivans (scar)	*Phlebotomus* *Phlebotomus*	*L. tropica major* *L. tropica minor* *L. aethiopica* (occasionally mucocutaneous) *L. infantum*
New World Mexico Brazil	Cutaneous Mucocutaneous (Chiclero ulcer) Espundia (mucosal) "beaked nose"	*Lutzomyia* *Lutzomyia* *Psychodopygus*	*L. mexicana,* *L. braziliensis species* *L. mexicana amazonensis* *L. b. braziliensis,* *L. b. Panamensis* (predilection for nose cartilage)
Visceral India America Mediterranean, etc.	Desert Storm patients Kala-azar	*Phlebotomus* *Lutzomyia* *Phlebotomus*	*L. tropica* *L. donovani* *L. d. chagasi* *L. infantum*
Disseminated cutaneous	Montenegro reaction negative		*L. aethiopica* (Old World) *L. mexicana complex* (New World)

[a] Diagnosis: Nicolle-Novy-MacNeal (NNN) medium, Giemsa and Wright stains, Montenegro skin test. Delayed-type hypersensitivity reaction is very specific.

[b] Treatment = IV sodium stibugluconate (need cardiac monitoring for T-wave flattening/inversion), topical paromycin, methylbenzothonium, emetine, methyl glutamine, ketoconazole, amphotericin B (good for resistant *L. donovani*), meglumine antimonate.

TABLE 4–20
LEPROSY REACTIONS

Reaction	Leprosy Type	Clinical Manifestations	After Therapy?	Immune Type	Treatment
Type 1	Borderline	Eruptive nodules in plaques, neuritis	Yes	Cell-mediated Th1	Steroids
Type 2	Borderline-lepromatous or Lepromatous leprosy	Erythema nodosum leprosy; eruptive nodules in normal skin	Yes	Immune complex Th2	Thalidomide
Lucio's phenomenon	Lepromatous leprosy	Vasculopathy, hemorrhage, bullae	No		Steroids (do not work)

TABLE 4–21
TREATMENT OF LEPROSY

Tuberculoid or Borderline leprosy	Borderline or borderline-lepromatous or lepromatous leprosy	One tuberculoid plaque = ROM
6 months: Rifampin 600 mg/ month, supervised Dapsone 100 mg/day	2 years: Rifampin 600 mg/month supervised Dapsone 100 mg/day Clofazimine 300 mg/ month, supervised ***OR*** clofazimine 50 mg/day, unsupervised	One-time dosage: **R**ifampin 600 mg **O**floxacin 200 mg **M**inocycline 100 mg

LYME VACCINE

- Remember that Lyme serologies cannot be relied on to confirm diagnosis (false + Lyme serology maybe due to treponemal disease, leptospirosis, relapsing fever, autoantibodies).
- 75% effective before infection; used in 15- to 70-year-olds in endemic areas (not pregnant).
- Vaccine = OspA; host antibodies to OspA kill *B. burgdorferi* (no other strain) in the tick, while the tick feeds.

TABLE 4–22
MARINE DERMATOSES

	Swimmer's Itch	Seabather's Eruption	Dogger Bank Itch
Etiology	*Schistosoma cercaria* (nonhuman schistosome)	*Cnidia larvae* (jellyfish = *Linuchae unguiculata*) *Edwardsiella lineate* = sea anemone larvae	*Alcyondium gelatonison*
Water	Fresh + salt (clamdigger's)	Salt	
Distribution	Uncovered areas	Covered areas	Eczematous dermatitis
Geography	North	South	North Sea

DIFFERENTIAL DIAGNOSIS OF MOLLUSCUM-LIKE LESIONS

- *Coccidioides*
- *Cryptococcus*
- *Penicillium marneffei*
- *Histoplasma*

TABLE 4–23
MYCETOMA (STAINS)

Type	PAS	Gram's	Fite's	Treatment
Eumycotic	+	–	–	
Botryomycotic (cocci)	–	+	–	
Actinomycotic (filament)	–	+	–	Penicillin G
Nocardial (filament)	–	+	+	Bactrim

MYCETOMA TRIAD

- Tumefaction (swelling)
- Draining sinus tracts
- Sulfur grains

TABLE 4–24
RUNYON CLASSIFICATION OF MYCOBACTERIA (ATYPICAL)

Group	Chromogen	Species	Pigment	Growth rate	Clinical Manifestations
1	PHOTO	*M. marinum* *M. kansasii*	Yellow after light exposure	2–3 weeks	Nodular lymphagitis
2	SCOTO	*M. scrofulaceum*	Yellow-orange	2–3 weeks	Neck
3	NON [[AU 27]]	*M. avium-intracellulare*	None	2–3 weeks	
		M. ulcerans			Buruli ulcer
4	Rapid growers	*M. fortuitum* *M. chelonei*	Variable	3–5 days	Wound infection use claithromycin

TABLE 4–25
MYCOSES (SYSTEMIC)

	Pathogenic	Opportunistic
Mycoses	Blasto-, coccidioido-, paracoccidioido-, histo-, and sporomycosis	*Aspergillus, Candida, Cryptococcus, Zygomyces*
Host defense	Normal	Compromised
Portal of entry	Pulmonary	Variable
Morphology	Dimorphic	Monomorphic
Distribution	Restricted	Ubiquitous

PARACOCCIDIOIDOMYCOSIS (SOUTH AMERICAN BLASTOMYCOSIS)

- Primary infection of the lungs.
- Secondary inoculation of mucous membranes and pharynx.
- Destructive facial lesions.
- Supraclavicular lymphadenopathy; appears like Hodgkin disease.
- Predisposition: after tooth extraction, picking teeth with twigs.
- Transformation from mycelial form to invasive yeast form inhibited by 17-beta-estradiol.
- Treatment: itraconazole (ketoconazole, amphotericin B).
- Bactrim for prophylaxis in HIV patients.

TABLE 4–26
DIFFERENTIAL DIAGNOSIS OF PARASITIZED MACROPHAGE[a]

Disease	Organism	Pathology (Inclusion Body)
HIStoplasmosis	*Histoplasma capsulatum*	Yeast with surrounding halo, scant lymphocytes
Granuloma **I**nguinale	*Calymmatobacterium granulomatis*	Donovan bodies ("safety pins"), lots of neutrophils
Rhinoscleroma	*Klebsiella rhinoscleromatis*	Mikulicz cell + Russell body, plasma cells
Leishmaniasis	*Leishmania*	Nucleus + kinetoplast, lymphocytes
Other		
Blastomycosis	*Blastomyces*	
Paracoccidio-idomycosis	*Paracoccidioidomyces*	
	Penicillium marneffei	
Trypanosomiasis	*Trypanosoma*	
Toxoplasmosis	*Toxoplasma*	

[a]Mnemonic: His girl.

PARVOVIRUS B19

Causes (ssDNA virus) the following:

- Erythema infectiosum (fifth disease): slapped cheeks appearance; then 3 weeks later, reticulate erythema on arms
- Aplastic anemia (crisis) in sickle cell patients
- Migratory polyarthritis in normal adults
- Thrombocytopenia in normal adults
- Hydrops fetalis (fetal death if infection of mother in first 20 weeks)
- Purpuric gloves-and-socks eruption (CD30 + T cells) (also seen with measles, coxsackie, CMV, and hepatitis B/EBV/HHV-6) (marker = pronormoblasts)

TABLE 4–27
PEDIATRIC INFECTIONS (CLASSIC SIX)

Disease	Names	Etiology	Clinical Manifestations
1	Rubeola = measles	Paramyxovirus	Rash, conjunctivitis, Koplik's spots (white) on buccal mucosa = altered sebaceous glands (not on palate)
2	Scarlet fever	*Streptococcus*	Sandpaper, white strawberry tongue, Pastia's petechial lines
3	Rubella = German measles	Togavirus	Deafness, cataracts, CHDs Earliest sign: patient has pain looking upwards + to the left Forscheimer's sign: Petechiae on soft palate + uvula
4	Filatow-Duke disease	Staph/strep	
5	Erythema infectiosum	Parvovirus B19	Slapped cheeks, reticular erythema
6	Exanthem subitum = roseola infantum	HHV-6	Morbilliform eruption, fever
	Gianotti-Crosti disease	EBV (US) Hepatitis B (Europe)	Erythematous papules on lower extremities, self-limited Forsheimer's spots: petechiae at soft/hard palate junction
	Haemophilus influenzae cellulitis	*H. influenzae*	Bluish plaque commonly seen on face

POXVIRUS

dsDNA, + cytoplasmic/intracytoplasmic inclusions
Pox

- Smallpox (variola)
- Vaccinia
- Molloscum
- Cowpox

Parapox

- Milker's nodule (pseudocowpox, paravaccinia)
- Orf disease

TABLE 4–28
RICKETTSIOSES

Disease	Species	Vector	Reservoir
Rocky Mountain Spotted fever (RMSF)	*Rickettsia rickettsii*	Rocky Mountain wood tick (*Dermacentor andersoni*) Eastern dog tick (*Dermacentor variabilis*)	Dogs, small animals
Rickettsialpox	*R. akari*	House mouse mite (*Allodermanyssus sanguineus*)	House mouse
Endemic typhus	*R. typhi*	Rat flea (*Xenopsylla cheopis*)	Rats
Epidemic typhus (Brill-Zinsser)	*R. prowazekii*	Human body louse (pediculosis corporis) Recrudescent; mild, resembles murine typhus	Flying squirrel, humans
Scrub typhus	*R. tsutsugamushi*	Chigger mite larva (*Eutrombicula hominis*)	Rodents
Boutonneuse fever	*R. conorii*	*Rhipicephalus sanguineus* dog tick	Dogs
• Sulfas contraindicated; RMSF first-line treatment is tetracyclines; second-line treatment is chloramphenicol			
Trench fever	*Bartonella quintana*	Human body louse	Humans
Q fever	*Coxiella burnetti*	Tick (*D. andersoni* + *Amblyomma americanum*)	Cattle, sheep, goats

TABLE 4–28
RICKETTSIOSES (*Continued*)

Disease	Species	Vector	Reservoir
Ehrlichiosis	*Ehrlichia chaffeensis*	Tick; causes leukocyte inclusions	Dogs
Leptospirosis	*Leptospira interrogans*	Fort Bragg + pretibial fever, Weil's disease	Dog/rat urine/tissue
Relapsing fever	*Borrelia recurrentis/ duttoni*	Human body louse + tick	Humans
Trench mouth	*Borrelia vincenti*	Vincent's angina: halitosis, gingival necrosis	
Noma	*Bacteroides* or *Borrelia*	Fusospirillary gangrenous stomatitis leads to rapid ulceration	

TABLE 4–29
DIFFERENTIAL DIAGNOSIS OF SPOROTRICHOID SPREAD

Deep Fungal	Bacterial	Other
Blastomycosis	Syphilis	Furunculosis
Coccidioidomycosis	Atypical mycobacteria	Leishmaniasis
Chromomycosis	Anthrax	
Histoplasmosis	Cat scratch	
Sporotrichosis	*Nocardia*	
	Francisella tularensis	

SPOROTRICHOSIS

- Common patients: miners (from supporting beams in mines).
- High temperature/humidity make infection more likely.
- Treatment: itraconazole, SSKI for cutaneous lymphonodular (not in pregnants).

TABLE 4–30
DISEASES MEDIATED BY STAPH/STREP TOXIN[a]

Disease	Etiology	Features
SSSS (Ritter disease)	Staph group 2 phage 71 (also bullous impetigo) and phage 55: produce exfoliative toxins A + B, which bind desmoglein 1	Neonates, desquamation, no oral lesion because no granular layer; NSAIDs contraindicated Nidus: nasopharynx, conjunctiva Predisposed by renal failure, immunosuppression, EtOH abuse, HIV disease, malignancy
TSS (staph) toxic shock syndrome	Staph phage 1: TSST-1 toxin Staph enterotoxins B + C (SEB, SEC) Superantigens that promote TNF-α, IL-1, IL-6	Perineal erythema, desquamation, strawberry tongue Tampons, nonmenstrual cases Nonmenstrual cases: i.e., nasal packing
TSS (strep) toxic shock syndrome	Group A strep M types 1,3: SPE = pyrogenic exotoxins A, B, C = superantigen	Preceded by soft tissue infection 80% of time; high mortality
REDD	Above	Recalcitrant erythematous desquamtive disorder = TSS in HIV
Scarlet fever	Strep pyogenes: pyrogenic exotoxins A, B, C	Sandpaper rash, Pastia's petechial lines, strawberry tongue, desquamation, glomerulonephritis

[a] Staph epidermidis causes thrombophlebitis in arm after intravenous line.

TABLE 4–31
SULFUR GRAINS

Mycetoma	Organism	Genus	Sulfur Grains
Eumycotic	Fungi	*Pseudallescheria, Madurella, Exophiala, Aspergillus, Acremonium*	Generally dark, except *Pseudallescheria, Aspergillus, Acremonium* = white
Actinomycotic	Gram$^+$ filamentous bacteria	*Actinomyces israelii* *Nocardia asteroides* (acid-fast) *Streptomyces*	Light *Actinomadura pelleteri* = red

TABLE 4–32
FINDINGS IN SYPHILIS

Stage	Findings		
Early congenital (before age 2)	Snuffles	Rhagades	Pemphigus = blisters/vesicles
	Dactylitis	Epiphysitis	Hepatitis
	Parrot's pseudoparalysis, secondary pain		
Late congenital (after age 2)	Keratitis (interstitial) → cataract	Saber shins	Clutton's joints (perisynovitis of knees)
	Mulberry molars	Saddle nose	Optic atrophy
	Hutchinson's teeth	Higoumanaki syndrome (clavicular fracture)	
	Hutchinson's triad (incisors, corneal opacities, eighth nerve deafness)		
Primary	Chancre (hunterian)	Redux = relapsed chancre	Dory flop
	Syphilis d'emblée	Edema indurativum = indurated edema + chancre	
	Balanitis of Follman: partially coalescent flat white papules on glans		

Secondary	Split papules	Papular	Corymbiform (ring of pustules)
	Pustular/ulcerative	Rupial = "oyster shell"	Lues maligna = pustules, fever, ulcer
	Alopecia	Mucous patch	Condyloma lata = most infectious
	Leukoderma colli	Annular	Pharyngitis
	Ollendorf sign -tender palmar papules		Meningitis
Tertiary	Noduloulcerative	Gummatous: most common location in oral cavity: tongue	
	Charcot joint = loss of contour	Paresis	Aortitis
	Argyll-Robertson pupil = accomodates but is unreactive to light		
	Tabes dorsalis: lose dorsal columns, neurotrophic ulcer, lose sensation: first temp, then pain, then touch		

JARISCH-HERXHEIMER REACTION

- Leptospirosis
- Relapsing fever (*Borrelia recurrentis;* louse-borne)
- Bacillary angiomatosis
- 6–8 h after penicillin treatment
- Mediated by TNF-α, IL-6

TABLE 4–33
BEST TESTS FOR SYPHILIS

Stage	Test	Other Information
Primary	FTA	RPR converts before VDRL
Secondary	Any (all +)	
Tertiary	FTA or MH-ATP	RPR or VDRL may be negative
Latent	MH-ATP better than FTA	

TABLE 4–34
TREATMENT OF SYPHILIS

Stage	First Line	Second Line	Third Line
HIV + primary syphilis	Penicillin G 2.4 million U/week × 3 weeks	None	None
Primary syphilis or secondary early latent <1 year	Penicillin G 2.4 million U × 1 week	Doxycycline × 2 weeks	Erythromycin[a] × 2 weeks
Secondary late latent or tertiary	Penicillin G 2.4 million U/week × 3 weeks	Doxycycline × 2–4 weeks	None
Neurosyphilis	Penicillin G 4 million U/4 h × 2 weeks, then 2.4 million U/week	None	None
Confirmed congenital	Penicillin G 100,000–150,000 μ/kg q12h × first 7 days of life, then q8h × 7–21 days of life	None[b]	None[b]
Unproven congenital	Penicillin G 50,000 μ/kg IM × 1 week	Procaine penicillin G 50,000 U IM/day × 2 weeks	None[b]

[a] Erythromycin not typically recommended.

[b] Pregnant and HIV patients should always be treated with penicillin G; if allergic, they should be desensitized and treated with penicillin G.

THERMODIMORPHIC FUNGI

Yeast at 37°C; hyphae at 25°C

- Blastomycosis
- Parracoccidiomycosis
- Histoplasmosis
- Sporotrichosis

TABLE 4–35
CAUSES OF DERMATOPHYTOSIS

Disease	Cause
Superficial white onychomycosis	Adults: *Trichophyton mentagrophytes* Children: *T. rubrum*
Tinea corporis	*T. rubrum* (most common), *T. mentagrophytes, M. canis*
Majocchi's granuloma	*T. rubrum* (secondary to tinea pedis)
Tinea pedis and manuum	*T. rubrum* (mocassin type) *T. mentagrophytes* (bullous) *Epidermophyton floccosum*
Tinea cruris (scrotum uninvolved)	*T. rubrum, E. floccosum*
Tinea barbae	*T. verrucosum, T. mentagrophytes*; spares upper lip
Tinea capitis	*T. tonsurans* (North America + western Europe) *T. violaceum* (eastern Europe)
Tinea versicolor	Yeast: *Pityrosporum obiculare*; Mold: *Malasezzia furfur* Mold: Occurs on penis only in immunosuppressed patients

TABLE 4–36
TREPONEMATOSIS (POSITIVE VDRL[[AU 40]])

Disease	Organism	Clinical Manifestations
Syphilis	*Treponema pallidum*	Bejel = endemic. Children exposed to syphilitic adults (saliva).
Pinta	*T. carateum*	South America. Hyperpigmentation, then depigmentation (no bone lesions).
Yaws	*T. pertenue*	Children: "mother" yaw (amber-crusted), then possibly bony lesions, then palmoplantar keratoderma. Spirochetes can be seen in tissue.

TABLE 4–37
TYPES OF TUBERCULOSIS

Contiguous = AFB+	Exogenous = AFB+	Hematogenous = AFB+	Tuberculids = PPD+, AFB–
Orificial	Verrucosis cutis	Miliary (PPD-)	Papulonecrotic (most common on extensor surfaces)
Scrofuloderma	Chancre	Gumma	Lichen scrofulorum
		Lupus vulgaris 10% AFB+	Erythema induratum

DIFFERENTIAL DIAGNOSIS OF UMBILICATED LESIONS

- Molluscum contagiosum
- Eczema herpeticum
- Smallpox/Variola
- Cryptococcus
- Histoplasmosis
- Coccidioidomycosis

VARICELLA VACCINE

- Live attenuated, 95% effective preventing severe episode, safe for people who have not been pregnant for 12 months
- HIV+ children may receive the vaccine as long as 25% of their T cells are CD4+

TABLE 4–38
VECTORS

Name	Species–Body Shape	Disease	Organism and Clinical Manifestations
Tick (*Ixodes, Dermacentor*)	*Ixodes dammini*; Northeast	Lyme disease	*Borrelia burgdorferi*
	I. scapularis; Northeast	Babesiosis	Waist-to-neck paralyzed
	I. pacificus; Southwest	Tick paralysis	
	I. racinus; Europe	Rocky Mountain spotted fever	
	Black legs, in ornate scutulum		
	D. variabilis; East	Ehrlichiosis	*Rickettsia ricketsii*
	D. andersoni; Rockies	Tick paralysis	*Ehrlichia chaffeensis*
	Brown legs, ornate scutulum	(Q fever) (Tularemia)	Above neck paralyzed
	Ambylomma americanum (lone star tick)	Tick paralysis	*Coxiella burnetti*
	Rhipicephalus sanguineus (dog tick)	Boutonneuse fever	*Francisella tularensis*
	Hard; eight legs		Waist down paralyzed
			R. conorii
Scabies mite	*Sarcoptes scabei*	Autofluoresces	Four legs in front, three in back
Chigger mite	Trombiculid red mite	Scrub typhus	*R. tsutsugamushi*
Eutrombicula hominae	Six legs with "spider body"	Tsutsugamushi fever	Kill chigger with DEET
House mouse mite	Allodermanyssus sanguineus	Rickettsialpox	*R. akari*
Head Louse	6 legs, large body	Pediculosis capitis	
Body louse	6 legs, large body	Typhus (epidemic)	*R. prowazekii*
	Pediculosis corporis ("Vagabond's disease")	Trench fever	*Bartonella quintana*
		Relapsing fever	*Borrelia recurrentis*

TABLE 4–38
VECTORS (*Continued*)

Name	Species–Body Shape	Disease	Organism and Clinical Manifestations
Pubic louse	Curved legs grab hair	"Crabs"	*Phthirus pubis* "Blue macules"
Sand fly "claws"	*Phlebotomus* (Old World) *Lutzomyia* (New World) Fat-winged mosquito	Leishmaniasis Bartonellosis (Oroya fever)	*Leishmania* species *B. bacilliformis*
Buffalo fly/black fly	*Simuliidae daminum* Overlapping wings, small head	Onchocerciasis River blindness: "hump" Fogo sevalgem	*Onchocerca volvulus* Mazotti reaction after DEC treatment
Deer or mango fly	*Chrysops* Regular-appearing fly with a yellow body	Loiasis ("Calabar swellings") (tularemia)	*Loa loa* = "eye worm" *F. tularensis*
Horsefly	*Tabanus*	Tularemia	*F. tularensis*
Tse tse fly	*Glossina* small = 1 mm; yellowish	African Trypanosomiasis "sleeping sickness"; Winterbottom sign = cervical LAN	*Trypanosoma rhodesiense* (acute) *T. gambiense* (chronic) blood smear shows worm structures
Myiasis/botfly Tumbu fly	Diptera larva *Dermatobia hominis*	Wound infection Furunculosis	Occasionally larva attaches to humans via mosquito bite
Bedbug	*Cimex lectularius* = fat bug		Flask-shaped eggs

Kissing bug	Reduviid: wings are crossed, thin cone nose, black with yellow color	American trypanosomiasis (Chagas disease)	*Trypanosoma cruzi romana* sign = unilateral lacrimal gland inflammation, conjunctivitis, eyelid edema 5 days after inoculation
Human flea Cat flea	*Pulex irritans* (no comb)[b] C. felis & C. canis (++comb) long legs, no wings	No disease except LE bites Bacillary angiomatosis Cat-scratch fever	*B. henselae*
Rat flea	*Xenopsylla cheopis* legs, no wings, ++comb	Plague Endemic typhus	*Yersinia pestis* *R. typhi*
Squirrel flea	*Diamanus montanus* legs, no wings, ++comb	Plague Endemic typhus	*Y. pestis* *R. typhi*
Water flea	Cyclops legs, no wings, ++comb	Guinea worm Sparganosis Larva migrans profundus	*Dracunculus medinensis* *Spirometra* Gnathostomiasis
Mosquito	*Anopheles/Aedes*[a] thin narrow wings	Filariasis Dirofilariasis Myiasis	*Wuchereria bancrofti* *Brugia malayi, B. timori* *Dirofilaria tenui, D. repens* *Dermatobia hominis*

[a] Mosquito attracted to humans by sweat and exhaled CO_2.
[b] Flea attracted to humans by displacement of air or vibrations.

TABLE 4–39
SEXUALLY TRANSMITTED DISEASES[a]

Disease	Organism	Best Diagnostic Test	First Line	Second Line
Chancroid	*Haemophilus ducreyi* (chocolate agar, school of fish) deep + ragged painful ulcer	Smear/culture (very difficult) if available, PCR or IIF (best)	Azithromycin	Ceftriaxone × 1 dose or erythromycin × 7 days or ciprofloxacin × 3 days
Chlamydia	*Chlamydia trachomatis*	Complement fixation titer < 1:16	Doxycycline	Erythromycin (pregnancy)
Gonorrhea (urethritis)	*Neisseria gonorrhoeae*	Urine culture	Ciprofloxacin × 1	Cefixime or Azithromycin
Gonococcemia	*N. gonorrhoeae*	Mucosal culture (best) or fluorescent antibody	Ceftriaxone IV	Ciprofloxacin or spectinomycin IV
Granuloma inguinale	*Calymmatobacterium granulomatis* (Caribbean: endemic) mildly tender ulcer	Smear (best): Giemsa or Wright stains: "safety pin" Donovan bodies. Biospy also OK	Bactrim or doxycycline × 3 weeks	Doxycycline or erythromycine × 3 weeks
Lymphogranuloma venereum	*Chlamydia trachomatis* Serotypes L1, L2, L3	Bubo aspirate culture (very difficult) or complement fixation titer > 1:64 (best)	Doxycycline × 3 weeks	Ciprofloxacin or erythromycin × 3 weeks
Lyme disease	*Borrelia burgdorferi*		Doxycycline	Amoxicillin (third = erythromycin)

[a] See also Tables 4–32 to 4–34 for information on syphilis.

[b] Gonococcemia occurs often 1 week after menses.

[c] In LGV, fibrosis may occur: esthiomene[[AU 45]](labia) or "saxophone" penis.

VIRUSES (DNA)

- Herpesvirus (HSV, CMV, EBV, VZV)
- Human papillomavirus (HPV)
- Adenovirus
- Poxvirus
- Parapoxvirus (Orf from sheep, milker's module caused by pseudocowpox and paravaccinia from cows)
- Parvovirus (single-stranded)

TABLE 4–40
VIRAL INCLUSION BODIES

Virus	Inclusion Bodies
Herpes	Lipschutz Electron microscopy: Cowdry type A
Smallpox/vaccinia	Guarnieri and Paschen
Molluscum contagiosum	Henderson-Patterson
HSV + HPV types	Intranuclear
Poxviruses	Intracytoplasmic
CMV	Both intranuclear and intracytoplasmic

TABLE 4–41
WORMS

Disease	Worm	Route/Clinical/Migration	Treatment
Amebiasis	*Entamoeba histolytica*	LE nodules, direct inoculation	Metronidazole
Cercarial dermatitis	Avian schistosome	Worm into skin, uncovered areas	Thorough washing
Bilharziasis (visceral Schistomosiasis)	*Schistosoma haematobium* (terminal *spine*) *S. mansoni* (lateral spine) *S. japonicum* (small spine)	Eggs into skin, bilharziomas Katayama (urticarial) fever	Praziquantel
Tapeworm/cysticercosis	*Taenia solium*	Ingest eggs; subcutaneous cysts; blood	Praziquantel
Tapeworm/sparganosis	*Spirometra*	Flesh poultice/ingest larva in cyclops	Excise or intralesional alcohol
Hydatid disease	*Echinococcus granulosus*	Ingest ova; subcutaneous cyst +liver/ lung disease	Excise or albendazole
Pinworm	*Enterobius vermicularis*	Ingest ova; anal pruritus; GI tract	Pyrantel pamoate, albendazole, or mebenda-zole
Hookworm	*Ancylostoma or Necator*	Larvae into feet; ground itch; GI tract	Mebendazole or albendazole
Larva migrans	*Ancylostoma brasiliensis*	Upper epidermis; Loeffler's syndrome: Lung infiltrates, 50% blood eosinophils, 90% sputum eosinophils	Topical thiabendazole, ivermectin or albendazole
Larva migrans profundus	*Gnathostoma doloris/ spinigerosa*	Ingest larval cyst (from raw flesh or cyclops flea); dermis	Excise +/– albendazole
Visceral larva migrans	*Toxocara canis*	Ingest eggs; pruritus, migrating panniculitis, eosinophils	DEC or thiabendazole
Larva currens	*Strongyloides stercoralis*	Ingest larva; perianal; intraepidermal fastest moving = cm/h	Ivermectin or albendazole

Guinea worm	*Dracunculosis midinensis*	Ingest larva in cyclops; subcutaneous induce worm extraction with water or ethyl chloride	Immerse in H_2O, excise, metronidazole (Flagyl)
Filariasis	*W. bancrofti, B. malayi;* see sheathed microfilariae in nighttime blood sample	Mosquito, lymphedema + tropical pulmonary eosinophilia, lymphatics	Ivermectin or DEC
Calabar swelling	*Loa loa*; see sheathed microfilariae in daytime blood sample	Chrysops fly, eye worm, blood, aspirate swellings for worms	DEC (reaction, occasionally encephalopathy, after ivermectin)
Onchocerciasis	*Onchocerca volvulus* see unsheathed microfilariae in skin snip	Black fly (larva); blindness; dermis (do skin snip)	Ivermectin (DEC → Mazotti) prednisone (eye involvement)
Dirofilariasis	*Dirofilaria tenuis/repens*	Mosquitos; red nodule; subcutaneous	Excise
Trichinosis	*Trichinella spiralis*	Ingest larval cyst, urticaria, splinter hemorrhage, paralysis; muscle	Albendazole, steroids (minimize reaction)
American trypanosomiasis (Chagas disease)	*Trypanosoma cruzi*	Reduviid bug; Romana sign, blood	Nifurtimox (with gamma-interferon)
African trypanosomiasis (sleeping sickness)	*T. rhodesiense* (acute) *T. gambiense* (chronic)	Tsetse fly; cercial lymphadenopathy; blood	Suramin, eflornithine (Vaniqa)
Streptocerciasis	*Mansonella streptocerca*	Lichen. papules + hypopigmented macules; skin snips = shepherd's crook	DEC

TABLE 4–42
WORMS: ROUTE OF TRANSMISSION

Ingest Larval Cyst	Ingest Ova	Ingest Larvae
Larva migrans profundus	*Cysticercus*	Larva currens
Trichinella spiralis	*Echinococcus*	Sparganosis
	Enterobius	Guinea worm (cyclops)

SECTION II

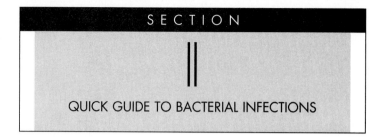

QUICK GUIDE TO BACTERIAL INFECTIONS

TABLE 4–43
GRAM-POSITIVE INFECTIONS

Infection	Organism	Treatment	Comments
Superficial pustular folliculitis (impetigo of Bockhart)	*Staphylococcus aureus*	1. Benzoyl peroxide or antibacterial soap 2. Hot compresses/Domeboro 3. Mupirocin ointment 2%	20% adults carry *S. aureus* in nares; HIV patients have twofold higher nasal carriage.
Sycosis vulgaris (barbae)	*S. aureus*	4. Penicillinase-resistant drug such as oxacillin, dicloxacillin 5. nasal carriage treated with 6. mupirocin	Tinea rarely infects upper lip. Pseudofolliculits manifests torpid papules.
Sycosis lupoides	*S. aureus*	7. PO dicloxacillin 8. PO rifampin 600 mg/day	Pustules with peripheral extension and central scar formation.
Furunculosis	*S. aureus*	9. cloxacillin 500 mg 4× daily or 10. low-dose clindamycin 150 mg/day × 11. 3 months 12. deeper abcesses need incision and drainage	Predisposition in diabetes, AIDS, EtOH, chronic granulomatous disease, dialysis, atopic dermatitis.
Carbuncles	*S. aureus*	13. for methicillin-resistant (MRSA): vancomycin	Two or more furuncles.
Pyogenic paronychia	*S. aureus, S. pyogenes, Pseudomonas, Proteus, Candida*	14. Penicillin allergy: clindamycin 15. If cultures show anaerobes, consider amoxicillin/clavulanate (Augmentin)	Subungual black macules in atopic dermatitis = osteomyelitis (get x-rays)
Botryomycosis	*S. aureus, Streptococcus, Pseudomonas, E. coli, Proteus, Bacteroides*	Antibiotics + excision	Sinuses discharge sulfur granules Diabetes, chronic granulomatous disease, Job's syndrome (hyper IgE syndrome), EtOH

Blastomycosis-like pyoderma			Verrucous, vegetative lesions with pustules
Pyomyositis	*S. aureus*	Incision, drainage, + antibiotics	Most commonly on thigh Need MRI to confirm diagnosis
Impetigo contagiosa	*S. aureus* (50–70%) (USA) Group A strep (developing nations) Group B strep (newborns)	Dicloxacillin or erythromycin (treat for 10 days if strep) For erythromycin resistance, Augmentin	If scalp involvement, check for pediculosis Acute glomerulonephritis: 1. 2–5% incidence under age 6 2. Group A strep by types 49, 55, 57, 60, and M type 2 3. Prognosis not affected by treatment May be early manifestation of HIV
Bullous impetigo (impetigo circinata)	*S. aureus,* group 2 page type 71, coagulase+		Neonatal type is highly contagious, Suggestive of pemphigus. Positive culture for *S. aureus* from the lesions.
Staphylococcal scalded skin syndrome (SSSS) (Ritter disease)	*S. aureus*, group 2 page type 71 (3A, 3B, 3C and 55) produce exfoliatin (exfoliative toxin)	Fluid resuscitation, systemic dicloxacillin	Take culture from mucous membranes, not lesions. In adults, check for renal failure or immunosuppression, less severe disease if exfoliatin cleared by kidneys.

TABLE 4–43
GRAM-POSITIVE INFECTIONS (*Continued*)

Infection	Organism	Treatment	Comments
Toxic shock syndrome (TSS)	*S. aureus* Strep M types 1 and 3, 80% produce exotoxin A (TSST 1, exotoxins B and C)	Nafcillin Incision and drainage Fluid resuscitation	Mortality of menstrual cases lower than of nonmenstrual. • Bulbar conjunctival hyperemia and palmar edema • Temperature of 38.9°C or higher • Erythematous eruption • Desquamation of palms/soles 1–2 weeks after onset • Hypotension • Three or more organ systems involved • Negative serologies: Rocky Mountain spotted fever, leptospirosis, rubeola • Negative PAN cultures
Ecthyma	Staph or strep	Mupirocin ointment, dicloxacillin	
Scarlet fever	Group A strep producing exotoxin	Penicillin, erythromycin, or cloxacillin	After strep pharyngitis, check throat swab and ASO titer Staph scarlatina without strawberry tongue Sandpaper quality papules on trunk Pastia's lines—linear petechiae over antecubital/axillae

			Desquamation of palms and soles Schultz-Carlton phenomenon—blanching due to antitoxin
Erysipelas (St. Anthony's fire)	Group A beta hemolytic strep Group B strep in newborns	Penicillin, erythromycin	Face and legs
Cellulitis	*S. aureus* *S. pyogenes*	First-generation cephalosporin Penicillinase-resistant penicillin	Needle aspirates of advancing edge 33 of 87 culture-positive 57% + if immunocompromised
Chronic lymphangitis	Staph/srep		Leads to chronic lymphangitis (elephantiasis nostras)
Necrotizing fasciitis	Beta-hemolytic strep, *Pseudomonas, Bacteroides*	Surgical debridement Antibiotics	Presence of anesthesia suggests deeper component "Probe test"; 20% mortality Poor prognosis in patients >50 years of age; in those with diabetes, delay of >7 days in diagnosis, infection on or near trunk
Blistering distal dactylitis	Group A beta-hemolytic strep *S. aureus*	PO antibiotics (penicillin)	Mainly toes, volar fat pad of phalanx Ages 2–16 typically affected; may occur in adults with diabetes

TABLE 4–43
GRAM-POSITIVE INFECTIONS (*Continued*)

Infection	Organism	Treatment	Comments
Perianal dermatitis	Group A strep, *S. aureus*	PO antibiotics (penicillin)	Throat cultures, perianal cultures; constipation in patients <8 years of age
	Group B strep (*S. agalactiae*)		Erysipelas, dactylitis, perianal dermatitis Sepsis and meningitis in neonates
Erysipeloid of Rosenbach	*Erysipelothrix rhusiopathiae* (rod shaped, gram +)	Self-limiting × 3 weeks Penicillin or erythromycin + rifampin	Swine, turkeys, saltwater fish/crabs Seen in meat-packers and fishermen; V-shaped filaments in culture
Pneumococcal cellulitis	*S. pneumoniae*	Penicillin	Blue/violaceous skin discoloration
Anthrax	Bacillus anthracis (rod-shaped, gram +) 1. Polyglutamic acid capsule 2. Edema toxin 3. Lethal toxin	Penicillin G IV × 6 days followed by PO penicillin × 10 days Tetracycline if penicillin-allergic	Necrosing painless carbuncle, suppurative adenitis Cutaneous, wool-sorter's disease and GI tract involvement Wool-sorters, cattlemen, tanners, butchers
Listeriosis	*Listeria monocytogenes* (gram + bacillus)	Ampicillin first line tetracycline, penicillin, erythromycin	Encephalitits/meningitis with monocytosis Serology better than culture

Leptospirosis 1. Weil disease 2. Fort Bragg fever	Many strains of *Leptospira* *L. interrogans* *L. autumnalis*	Tetracycline and penicillin Doxycycline 200 mg/week if traveling in endemic area	Sources: dogs, rats Icteric (Weil): chills, fever, icterus, purpura, azotemia Nonicteric (Fort Bragg fever): exanthem on shins, fever conjunctival injection Dark-field exam for spirochetes, guinea pig inoculation Serologies in the second week (IgM)
Diptheria	*Corynebacterium diptheriae* (Klebs-Loeffler bacillus)	Diphtheria antitoxin (rule out hypersensitivity to horse serum via conjunctival test) Erythromycin Rifampin for carrier state IV penicillin G for severe cases	1. ulcer with leathery, grayish membrane 2. eczematous/pustular (+ for *C. diptheriae*) Postdiphtheria paralysis and cardiac complications

TABLE 4–44
BACTERIAL INFECTION ASSOCIATED WITH ULCERS

Infection	Organism	Treatment	Comments
Desert sore (Barcoo rot)	*C. diptheriae*, staph and strep	Diphtheria antitoxin Oral penicillin or erythromycin	Bushmen in Australia and soldiers in Burma Grouped vesicles become ulcers
Tropical ulcer	*Borrelia vincentii, Bacterodies fusiformis*		Scratch to inflammatory papules to ulcers (extremities)
Septic desert ulcer	*C. diptheiae*		
Gummatous punched-out ulcer	*Treponema pallidum*		
Tuberculous ulcer	*M. tuberculosis*		Undermined, usually not on the LE
Frambesia ulcer	*Treponema pertenue*		
Buruli ulcer	*M. ulcerans*		

CORYNEBACTERIAL INFECTIONS

Infection	Organism	Treatment	Comments
Erythrasma	*Corynebacterium minutissimum*	Erythromycin PO or top Topical miconazole or clindamycin	Coproporphyrin III results in coral-red fluorescence
Pitted keratolysis	*Corynebacterium, Micrococcus sedentarius*	Topical erythromycin or clindamycin 5% Benzoyl peroxide gel	Malodorous; affecting weight-bearing part of sweaty feet
Trichomycosis axillans	*Corynebacterium tenuis*		Concretions on hair shafts

TABLE 4–45
GANGRENE

Infection	Organism	Treatment	Comments
Gas gangrene	*Clostridium perfringens* (thick gram + rods)	Surgical debridement, IV penicillin G, and hyperbaric oxygen	Differential diagnosis of crepitus: 1. *Clostridium* (*perfringens, septicum*, hemolyticum) 2. *Streptoccus* (*fecalis, anginosus*) 3. *Proteus, Bacteroides, Escherichia coli, Klebsiella*
Chronic undermining, burrowing ulcers (Meleney's gangrene)	*Peptostreptococcus* *S. aureus, Enterobacter*	Triple antibiotics including penicillin, aminoglycosides	Postoperative gangrene
Fournier's gangrene	Group A strep Enteric bacilli/anaerobes	Debridement Antibiotics	Penis and scrotum, ages 20–50 mainly

TABLE 4–46
GRAM-NEGATIVE INFECTIONS

Infection	Organism	Treatment	Comments
Ecthyma gangrenosum	*Pseudomona aeruginosa*	Double coverage (aminoglycoside and piperacillin)	Debilitated patients (leukemia, burns, chronic granulomatous disease, neutropenic, cancer) Starts as a vesicle, hemorrhagic pustule Assume pseudomonal sepsis; systemic therapy
Green nail syndrome	*P. aeruginosa*	Benzoyl peroxide or 1% acetic acid soaks, debridement	Onycholysis
Gram-negative toe web infection	*P. aeruginosa* *E. coli, Proteus*	Treat for dermatophytosis May need systemic antibiotics	Begins with dermatophytosis Consider swab for culture if intertrigo nonresponsive to antifungals
Blastomycosis-like pyoderma	*P. aeruginosa, S. aureus*	Ciprofloxacin	
Hot-tub folliculitis	*P. aeruginosa*	Self-limiting; 7–14 days If systemic symptoms, ciprofloxacin	Appears 1–4 days after soaking in hot tub Chlorination of water, pH 7.2–7.8 Malignant external otitis (facial nerve palsy in 30%)

TABLE 4–47
MISCELLANEOUS INFECTIONS

Infection	Organism	Treatment	Comments
Malakoplakia	*P. aeruginosa, E. coli, S. aureus*	Based on organism isolated ciprofloxacin/ofloxacin, trimethoprim/sulfamethoxazole (Bactrim), penicillin, clofazamine, bethanecol	Granuloma of GU tract, skin affected in immunocompromised patients Foamy eosinophilic Hansemann macrophages with calcified, concentric Michaelis-Gutmann bodies
Chancroid	*Haemophilus ducreyi* (gram–bacillus)	First line: azithromycin × 1 dose erythromycin, ceftriaxone, ciprofloxacin Avoid ciprofloxacin in patients <17 years of age and in pregnant patients	Tender genital ulcers, unilateral painful adenitis, M > F Phagedena: spreading/sloughing ulceration Check HIV and RPR (HIV transmission facilitated)
Granuloma inguinale (donovanosis)	*Calymmatobacterium granulomatis* (gram–)	Bactrim × 3 weeks or until healed Ciprofloxacin or erythromycin base Use IV gentamycin if lesions are nonresponsive	Painless serpiginous groin ulcers Esthiomene: pseudoelephantiasis of genitals Ulcers complicated by sinus tracts and SCC in women >20 μm macrophages with Donovan bodies seen by silver or Giemsa staining, or toluidine blue staining
Gonococcemia	*Neisseria gonorrhoeae*	Ceftriaxone IV × 48 h, then cephalosporins Spectinomycin if patient is allergic to beta-lactams Ciprofloxacin and ofloxacin provide good prophylaxis in single doses, ceftriaxone IM × 1	Fever, hemorrhagic pustules, monoarticular involvement Consider C5, C6, C7, or C8 deficiency if using cephalosporins alone, add tetracycline to cover chlamydia

TABLE 4–47
MISCELLANEOUS INFECTIONS (*Continued*)

Infection	Organism	Treatment	Comments
Meningococcemia	*Neisseria meningitidis* (gram–diplococcus)	Penicillin G IV 4 million U four times daily × 7 days Chloramphenicol in penicillin-allergic Rifampin 600 mg × 2 days (to clear nasal carriage and treat if exposed)	Present with fever, chills, hypotension and meningitis 50–65% of patients with petechiae/purpura chronic variant, recurrent fever and rash, human nasal carriage 5–10% Polyvalent vaccine effective against groups A, C, Y, W-135 Waterhouse-Friderichsen syndrome: adrenal hemorrhage Shwartzman phenomenon
Vibrio vulnificus infection	*V. vulnificus* (noncholera, gram–rod)	First line: doxycycline + ceftazidime Penicillin, cephalosporins, tetracycline, cotrimoxazole	Raw oyster ingesion, sea-water aspiration, cutaneous entry Hemorrhagic bullae, petechiae, purpura Risk factors: chronic liver disease, immunosuppression, diabetes, EtOH, hemochromatosis, renal failure
Salmonellosis	*Salmonella typhi* (gram–rods)	Ceftriaxone or fluoroquinolone	Rose spots in 50–60% of cases; erythema typhosum Poultry products, contaminated food and water Blood, stool, and bone marrow cultures
Rhinoscleroma	Klebsiella pneumoniae, K. rhinoscleromatis (gram–rod)	Fluoroquinolones + steroids Ciprofloxacin is first-line therapy Surgical correction of deformities	Chronic granulomatous disease of upper respiratory tract Extensive mutilation

			Mikulicz's cells (Frisch bacilli with silver stain) Russell bodies (Ig in degenerated plasma cells)
Pasteurellosis	*Pateurella hemolytica* *P. multocida* (gram–rods)	Penicillin or tetracycline	Pathogen of domestic animals Injuries from animal bites
Dog bites	*Capnocytophaga canimorsus* (DF-2 gram–rod) Eugonic fermenting bacteria (EF-4)	Trimethoprim/sulfamethoxazole (Augmentin)	Splenectomized patients at risk for: 1. DF-2 2. *H. influenzae* group B 3. Babesiosis 4. *N. meningitidus* 5. Group A strep
Human bites	*Eikenella corrodens* (gram–rods)	Trimethoprim/sulfamethoxazole (Augmentin)	Human bites or fistfights
Glanders	*Pseudomonas mallei*	Streptomycin + tetracycline	Horses, mules or donkeys; nasal discharge/epistaxis Inflammatory papule that ulcerates, then "farcy buds" (nodules along lymphatics)
Melioidosis (Whitmore disease)	*Burkholderia pseudomallei*	Tetracycline and trimethoprim/sulfamethoxazole (Augmentin), third-generation cephalosporins	Pulmonary and septicemic forms Subcutaneous and multiple sinuses of soft tissues

TABLE 4–47
MISCELLANEOUS INFECTIONS (*Continued*)

Infection	Organism	Treatment	Comments
Cat-scratch disease	*B. henselae*	Self-limiting Erythromycin, tetracycline, or doxycycline, azithromycin	Cat to cat by fleas and cat to human by scratches Most frequent cause of chronic LAN in children/young adults Serology negative early in the disease Skin testing (Hanger and Rose test) can be used
Bacillary angiomatosis	*B. henselae* (lymph node, liver, spleen) *B. quintana* (bone, subcutaneous mass)	Erythromycin or doxycycline prophylactic regimens include erythromycin or rifampin	Jarisch-Herxheimer reaction may occur with first dose CD4 cells usually <50/mL Can occur in immunocompetent hosts Lesions resemble pyogenic granulomas
Trench fever	*B. quintana*	Ceftriaxone followed by erythromycin	Associated with body louse infestation Fevers that lasts a week, then recurs in 5 days; endocarditis
Oroya fever + Verruca peruana	*B. bacilliformis* (transmitted by *Lutzomyia verrucarum*)	Chloramphenicol (*Salmonella* coinfection common)	Oroya fever with hemolytic anemia, leukopenia Untreated fatality is 40–88%, treated is 8% Then eruptive verruga peruana occurs (heals with no scarring) Bacteria within/attached to erythrocytes (Giemsa)

TABLE 4–49
TYPHUS GROUP

Infection	Organism	Treatment	Comments
Endemic typhus (murine)	*Rickettsia typhi* (transmitted by *Xenopsylla cheopis*)	Doxycycline in single dose Vaccination and delousing	Murine infection OX-19 test positive
Epidemic typhus (louse-borne)	*Rickettsia prowazekii* (transmitted by *Pediculus humanus* var. *corporis*)	Same as endemic typhus	Gangrene of fingers, toes, ears may occur 6–30% mortality OX-19 positive after 8–12 days Brill-Zinsser disease (recurrence) like murine typhus

TABLE 4–50
SPOTTED FEVER GROUP

Infection	Organism	Treatment	Comments
Rocky Mountain spotted fever	*Rickettsia rickettsii* Wood tick = *D. andersoni* Dog tick = *D. variabilis* Lone star tick = *Amblyomma americanum*	Tetracycline 25–50 mg/kg/day, chloramphenicol	Ankles, wrists with petechial eruption *R. rickettsii* present in initial rash on IF testing OX-2 and OX-19 positive in second week of illness Nephritis is main complication
Boutonneuse fever (Mediterranean fever)	*R. conorii* Dog tick = *Rhipicephalus sanguineus*	Good prognosis without therapy Tetracycline or chloramphenicol	OX-2 and OX-19+ Tick bite produces indurate papule = tache noir
Rickettsialpox	*R. akari* Rodent mite = *Allodermanyssus sanguineus*	Self-limiting in 2 weeks Tetracycline	Mus musculus (house mouse is reservoir) Prevalent in New York City; direct fluorescent antibody of eschar Weil Felix test negative
Scrub typhus (tsutsugamushi fever)	*R. tsutsugamushi* (trombiculid red mite = chigger)	Tetracycline	Antibody to OX-K occur in 50% by second week (cross-react with lepto) Deafness or tinnitus occur in 20% untreated cases
Ehrlichiosis	*Ehrlichia chaffeensis*	Tetracycline	30% with eruption

TABLE 4–51
BORRELIA

Infection	Organism	Treatment	Comments
Lyme disease	*B. burgdorferi* (USA) *B. garinii* (Europe) *B. afzelii* (Europe) *Ticks (Ixodidae):* *Ixodes scapularis* (Northeast/Midwest) *I. pacificus* (West) *I. ricinus* (Europe)	Doxycycline 200 mg/day for 10–30 days *Children <9 years:* amoxicillin 20 mg/day *Pregnant patients:* 1. localized/early = amoxicillin 2. disseminated = penicillin G *Arthritis/Meningitis/Cardiac:* 1. Ceftriaxone 2 g/day × 2 weeks 2. IV penicillin G (50% nonresponders)	Tick must be attached for 24 h for transmission “moving freckle” prophylactic antibiotics after tick bite not recommended Transplacental transmission has been documented “Banworth syndrome” = focal, severe radicular pains, lymphocytic meningitis, cranial nerve paralysis when erythema migrans present alone, 67% + ELISA 60–80% get erythema migrans; chronic arthritis occurs in the knees
Acrodermatitis chronica atrophicans	*B. afzelii* (transmitted by *I. ricinus*)	Penicillin G or doxycycline	Also known as “primary diffuse atrophy”; “ulnar bands” = well-defined, smooth, band-like thickenings from finger to elbow or shins Warthin-Starry positive in some cases

TABLE 4–52
OTHER MISCELLANEOUS BACTERIAL INFECTIONS

Infection	Organism	Treatment	Comments
Plague	*Yersinia pestis* (gram–bacillus) (transmitted by *Xenopsylla cheopis*)	First line: streptomycin, kanamycin, chloramphenicol, tetracycline	Bubonic plague (89% Rocky Mountains)
Rat bite fever	*Spirillum minus* *Streptobacillus moniliformis* (gram–rod)	Cauterization of bite by nitric acid Tetanus propylaxis, penicillin × 3 days	1. "soduko" by *S. minus* 2. septicemia by *S. moniliformis* (Haverhill fever)
Tularemia	*Francisella tularensis* (gram–coccobacillus) (transmitted by *Dermacentor andersonii* or *Amblyomma americanum*)	Streptomycin × 10 days Gentamicin Tetracycline in doses >2 g/day × 15 days	1. Ulceroglandular type, ulceration with sporotrichoid spread, fever, examthem 2. Typhoidal type, fever, malaise, GI symptoms 3. Oculoglandular type
Brucellosis (undulant fever)	*Brucella abortus* (gram–rods)	Doxycycline + rifampin erythromycin or tetracycline for 6–8 days	Contact with infected animals and animal products
Mycoplasmal infection	*Mycoplasma pneumoniae*		Not viruses or bacteria Stevens-Johnson syndrome most frequent complication, erythema multiforme Cold agglutinin titer >1:128 to make diagnosis

TABLE 4–53
CHLAMYDIA

Lymphogranuloma venereum	*Chlamydia trachomatis* (L1, L2, L30)	Doxycycline erythromycin (treat partners)	Suppurative inguinal lymphadenopathy Starts with a herpetiform ulcer that heals 2 weeks later, enlargement of regional lymph nodes ("groove sign") Esthiomene may occur

CHAPTER 5

TUMORS

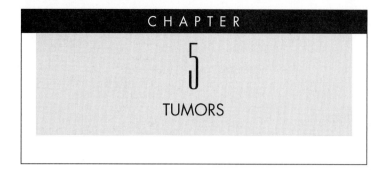

TABLE 5–1
ADNEXAL TUMORS

Lesion	Clinical or Pathologic Finding
Accessory nipple	Invaginated pilosebaceous unit underlying glands + muscle; "milk line"
Adenoid cystic carcinoma/ eccrine epithelioma	Scalp; perineural invasion; similar to Microcystic adrenal carcinoma (MAC)
Chrondroid syringoma (mixed tumor)	Most common site is head + neck; pseudocartilaginous, lace-like patterns of pale blue cells, ducts, mucinous stroma
Cylindroma	Jigsaw puzzle; scalp
Dermal duct tumor	Monomorphic big blue balls (like poroma), with small ducts only in dermis (see hidroacanthoma, below)
Desmoplastic trichoepithelioma	Depressed center; syringoma-like with horn cysts, fibrovascular stroma, focal calcification
Eccrine hidrocystoma	Seasonal variation, eyelids
Eccrine poroma	Monomorphic blue tumor with small ducts extending from epidermis (dermal duct, hidroacanthoma)
Eccrine spiradenoma	Painful; overlying skin blue; blue balls in dermis with ductal differentiation, alveolar pattern
Eccrine syringo-fibroadenoma	Anastomosing epithelial strands surrounded by fibrous stroma; "hamburger" meat appearance
Fibrofolliculoma	Cystically dilated follicle, proliferation of outer root sheath epithelium + perifollicular fibrosis
Hidradenoma papilliferum	Vulva; epithelial papillae, usually no epidermal component

TABLE 5–1
ADNEXAL TUMORS (*Continued*)

Lesion	Clinical or Pathologic Finding
Hidroacanthoma simplex	Acanthotic epidermis, intraepidermal monomorphic blue cells with small ducts (see poroma, dermal duct, below)
Malignant chondroid syringoma	Metastases may have minimal chondroid component
Microcystic adnexal carcinoma	Upper lip, high local recurrence; appears like a deep invasive syringoma
Nevus sebaceous	Apocrine glands notable in adult biopsy. Infant biopsy: sebaceous glands at epidermis
Nodular hidradenoma/ eccrice acrospiroma	Blue balls in dermis with cystic degeneration, clear cell change
Papillary eccrine adenoma	Blacks, females, legs; dermal cystically dilated ducts with epithelial processes
Pilar (trichilemmal) cyst	Basal cell layer, squamous layer, no granular layer, homogenous eosinophilic contents
Pilar sheath acanthoma	Upper lip, widened pore with invagination
Pilomatricoma	Shadow cells, blue cells, hard nodule, younger patients, calcification
Porocarcinoma	Cutaneous (epidermotropic metastases)
Proliferating trichilemmal like, no shadow	Scalp, Squamous cell carcinoma (SCC)-tumor cells, lobular growth
Sebaceous carcinoma	Eyelids, in situ pagetoid spread
Steatocystoma	Females, eyelids, Down syndrome
Syringocystadenoma papilliferum	Invagination from epidermis, double-layered epithelial papillae, apocrine glands; plasma cells
Syringoma	Corrugated lining, sebaceous glands
Trichoadenoma	Numerous dermal keratin cysts, fibrovascular stroma
Trichodiscoma	Raised papule, lateral collarette, fibrous proliferation in dermis
Trichoepithelioma	Palisaded blue balls with horn cysts, papillary mesenchymal bodies, no retraction
Trichofolliculoma	Tuft of hair; well-developed dilated follicle surrounded by multiple smaller follicles
Trichilemmoma	Warty, acanthosis with clear glycogen filled keratinocytes
Tumor of the follicular infundibulum	Plate-like growth of follicular epithelium
Vellus hair cyst	Thin-walled, many vellus hairs

TABLE 5–2
TYPES OF ANGIOSARCOMA

Classic	Elderly (head + neck) factor VIII+; sudden thrombocytopenia sign of metastatic disease, bruise with peripheral satellite nodules; Stuart-Treves secondary to chronic lymphedema, >10 yr after surgery. Poor prognosis without early amputation; metastatic to lungs. Site of prior x-ray therapy (many years after).
Dabska's	Low-grade, occurs in infants
Retiform hemangioendothelioma	Low-grade, occurs in young adults

TABLE 5–3
BASAL CELL CARCINOMA

Treatment Modality	Cure Rate
Electrodessication and cutterage (ED + C)	>90% (nonmorpheaform, nonfacial)
Excision	95% with 4-mm margins
Mohs	99% (primary), 96% (recurrent)

CARCINOID

- Elevated 5-hydroxyindolacetic acid (5-HIAA) in 24-h urine: 3–8 mg is normal; >25 mg is diagnostic.
- Banana pulp, tomatoes, plums, avocadoes, eggplant can increase 5-HIAA.
- Screening test: use nitrosonaphthol, which turns urine purple if 5-HIAA > 40 mg in 24-h urine.
- Treatment: remove tumor, 5-FU, decrease tryptophan-containing foods, IV octreotide + streptozocin.
- Associated with MEN type I, generalized hyperhidrosis, pellagra-like eruption.

DIFFERENTIAL DIAGNOSIS OF CD30+ LYMPHOMA

- Lymphomatoid papulosis
- CTCL (large cell anaplastic type)
- Hodgkin disease (Reed-Sternberg cells)

PROGNOSIS OF CD30 + LESION

- Solitary nodule = favorable prognosis
- Extracutaneous (i.e., lymph node) = poor prognosis
- CD30 − CTCL transforming into CD30+ cells = poor prognosis

CHLOROMA

- Granulocytic sarcoma (congenital leukemia)
- Green color is from myeloperoxidase

METASTATIC RATES OF DERMATO FIBRO SARCOMA PROTUBERANS (DFSP)

- Overall: 3%
- Recurrence rate with conventional surgery: 49%
- Recurrence with 3-cm margins: 11%
- Recurrence with Mohs: unknown

FOLLICULAR B-CELL LYMPHOMA

- CD10+
- M > F
- M: trunk, good prognosis, CD10+, bcl-2−
- F: legs: bad prognosis, CD10+, bcl-2+

FOLLICULAR MUCINOSIS

- face biopsy with eosinophils, mucin present
- treat with PUVA, steroids

GLOMUS TUMOR

- Hands/feet, especially subungual
- Solitary (tender), multiple (nontender) → can lead to glomangiosarcoma
- Sucquet-Hoyer canal stains with vimentin (smooth muscle cells)

TABLE 5–4
MARKERS OF HISTIOCYTOSIS

DISEASE	S-100	CD1a	Birbeck	Mϕ/CD68	Prognosis	Age
Histiocytosis X	+	+	++	–	↓	↓
Congenital self-healing (Hashimoto-Pritzker)	+	+	+ (10–25%)	–	↓	↓
Indeterminate cell (dermal dendrocytes)	+	occ+	–	+	↓	↓
Sinus histiocytosis (Rosai-Dorfman)[a]	+	–	–	+	↓	↓
Non-X histiocytosis[b]	–	–	–	+	Better	Older

[a] Some authors: Rosai-Dorfman is CD1a positive.
[b] Histiocytosis X is also ATPase-positive.

TABLE 5–5
TYPES OF HISTIOCYTOSIS

Disease	Characteristics
Letterer-Siewe	Mucosal,seborrheic dermatitis-like, nail changes, hepatosplenomegaly, osteolysis (skull/cranium)
Hand-Schuller-Christian	Diabetes insipidus, bone lytic lesions (map-like), exophthalmos, one-third with skin changes
Eosinophilic granuloma	Localized osteolysis: cranium, ribs, vertebrae, pelvis; eosinophilic
Hashimoto-Pritzker	Congenital self-healing reticulohistiocytosis: head, neck, trunk, proximal extremities (no mucosal lesions)
Benign cephalic histiocytosis	Pediatric, head + neck, multiple lesions, self-involute
Rosai-Dorfman	Fever, increasing ESR, leukocytosis, polyclonal hypergammaglobulinemia 90%
Pathology	Giant cells with ground-glass cytoplasm, wreathlike nuclei

INFANTILE DIGITAL FIBROMATOSIS

- Benign; spares thumb and big toe
- 47% in first month of life
- Eosinophilic lamellar inclusions: made of actin (stain +)
- Stains: actin-specific enolase, Masson trichome (red), phosphotungstic acid hematoxylin (PTAH=purple)
- Myofibromatosis—most common fibrous tumor of infancy

INFANTILE FIBROMATOSIS

- *Diffuse:* affects muscles of arms, neck, and shoulders
- *Aggressive:* fast-growing lesions in first year, limbs/trunk, appear malignant on pathology
- *Congenital generalized:* multiple dermal nodules may resolve within 2 years, 80% mortality due to vital organ compression, good prognosis if patient survives 4 months
- *Fibrous hamartoma of infancy:* one truncal lesion, cell-poor fibrous lesion

JUVENILE XANTHOGRANULOMA

1. *Clinical:* “pumpkin” color
2. *Ocular:* glaucoma > anterior chamber hemorrhage (hyphema) > retinal detachment > heterochromic irides
    - Eye problems occur in <1% (iris lesions > eyelid lesions)
    - More than three lesions = higher likelihood of eye problems

3. *Systemic:* eye (iris) > lung > liver
4. *Associated conditions:* NF-1, juvenile chronic myelogenous leukemia, aquagenic pruritus
5. *Differential diagnosis:* histiocytosis X, congenital self-healing, benign cephalic, mastocytoma, Spitz nevus
6. *Pathology*: histiocytes, Touton giant cells
7. *Immunohistochemistry:* Positive—CD68, factor XIIIa, HAM56; Negative—S-100, MAC 387

KAPOSI SARCOMA

1. *Classic:* Mediterranean, East European on lower extremities, soft palate, lymphedema, may involute spontaneously
2. *African cutaneous:* vascular masses on extremities, locally aggressive, males
3. *African lymphadenopathic:* lymph node changes with/without cutaneous manifestations; patients die within 2 years
4. HIV disease can be fatal; cutaneous + visceral manifestations
5. *Kaposi sarcoma with lymphoma:* similar to classic except that site of lesions varies
   - GI tract most frequently involved organ, small intestine most common
   - Bony changes signal widespread disease
   - Poses 20 times higher risk of lymphoreticular malignancy
   - Associated with HHV-8
6. Treatment: Less than 10 new lesions per month lead to x-ray therapy, excision, alitretinoin gel, intralesional vincristine; more than 10 new lesions per month or symptomatic lymphedema/pulmonary disease leads to systemic treatment (actinomycin D, interferon, vinblastine)

CLINICAL TYPES OF KERATOACANTHOMA

Involucrin stains homogenously (SCC stains irregularly).
Solitary

- Giant
- KA centrifugum marginatum
- Subungual Multiple (associated with immunosuppression and SLE-eruptive)
- Multiple self-healing (Ferguson-Smith)
- Eruptive (Grzybowski)

TABLE 5–6
MELANOMA: EXCISION MARGINS AND SURVIVAL RATE[a]

Breslow Depth (mm)	Margin (cm)	Survival Rates (5-and 10-year)
<1	1	90–99%
1–2	1–2	75–90%
2–4	2	60–75%
>4	3	<50%

[a] Nodular ulcerated (unrelated to depth), 60–70%.

TABLE 5–7
STAGING AND TREATMENT OF MELANOMA[a]

Stage	Disease Characteristics	Treatment
Stages 1 + 2	Local disease	Excise (> 1 mm thick = sentinel lymph node)
Stage 3	Regional lymph node or in-transit metastases (>2 cm from primary tumor)	IFN-α_{2B}
Stage 4	Distant disease (beyond local lymph nodes)	IL-2, dacarbazine, melphalan

[a] Giant congenital nevi: 8% risk of developing malignant melanoma.

METASTATIC SITES OF MELANOMA

- 60% appear in skin, subcutis, lymph nodes
- 36% lungs
- 20% liver
- 20% brain
- 17% bone
- 11% GI tract

MERKEL CELL CARCINOMA

- Excision requires at least 3-cm margins
- Chemotherapy includes intralesional TNF-α
- 44% of patients have head and neck metastasis

SKIN METASTASES: MOST COMMON PRIMARIES

Women	Men
1. Breast 2. Lung 3. Colon	1. Lung 2. Colon 3. Melanoma

MULTICENTRIC RETICULOHISTIOCYTOSIS

- Red-brown nodules: seen on face, hands, arms, scalp, neck, mucous membranes
- Arthritis mutilans
- 28% of cases are paraneoplastic

MULTIPLE MYELOMA: ASSOCIATIONS

- Follicular spicules on nose
- Leukocytoclastic vasculitis
- Ichthyosiform dermatitis
- Raynaud's phenomenon

- Alopecia
- Primary systemic amyloid
- Plantar palmar xanthomas
- Necrobiotic xanthogranuloma

NECROBIOTIC XANTHOGRANULOMA

- Face > trunk > extremities. Periorbital ~85%
- Red-orange nodules become centrally ulcerated
- Cholesterol clefting, Touton giant cells, central necrobiosis with palisading foamy giant cells
- Associations: paraproteinemia, multiple myeloma, IgG-Kappa chain, primary biliary cirrhosis
- Extracutaneous: eye number-one site = orbital mass

NODULAR FASCIITIS

Onset age 40, sudden appearance, + tender
Childhood variant = craniofasciitis that may invade the cranium

PAGET DISEASE (EXTRAMAMMARY)

- Most common site in descending order: vulva, perianal area, penis, scrotum
- May present as perianal lichenified plaque

MNEMONIC FOR DIFFERENTIAL DIAGNOSIS OF PAINFUL TUMORS

Blend an egg:

Blue rubber bleb nevus syndrome	• Cavernous hemangioma in dermis
Leiomyoma	• Pain with cold; spindle cells: pilar, angio, dartus (genital, no pain)
Eccrine spiradenoma	• Blue islands, two cell types, similar to cylindroma
Neuroma	• Nerves with fibrosis
Dercum's adiposis	• Pararticular; can be treated with IV lidocaine
Dolorosa dermatofibroma	
Angiolipoma/angioleiomyoma	
Neurilemmoma/Schwannoma	• Antoni A areas (Verocay bodies) and Antoni B areas
Endometriosis	• Usually periumbilical with perimenstrual bleeding apparent
Glomus tumor	• Actin+, hands/feet (nails); glomangioma usually not painful
Granular cell tumor	• Tongue 40%, usually S-100+

NEOPLASMS ASSOCIATED WITH PARANEOPLASTIC PEMPHIGUS

In order of decreasing frequency:

1. Non-Hodgkin lymphoma
2. Chronic lymphocytic leukemia (CLL)
3. Castleman disease (HHV-8)
4. Sarcoma (poorly differentiated)

5. Thymoma
6. Waldenstrom's macroglobulinemia
7. Fibrosarcoma (inflammatory)
8. Bronchogenic SCC
9. Round-cell liposarcoma
10. Hodgkin disease
11. T-cell lymphoma

MNEMONIC FOR SOLITARY RED BUMP
Space:

Spitz nevus
Pyogenic granuloma
Amelanotic melanoma
Clear cell acanthoma
Eccrine poroma
Merkel cell tumor
Cutaneous metastasis

TYPES OF SEBORRHEIC KERATOSIS

- Acanthotic
- Hyperkeratotic
- Adenoidal (reticulated)
- Clonal
- Inflamed (irritated or inverted follicular)
- Melanoacanthoma (pigmented)

SÉZARY SYNDROME

1. Erythroderma
2. Lymphadenopathy
3. Atypical cells on peripheral smear
   (normal smear: CD4 = 35–55%, CD8 = 19–32%, and CD7 = 58–74%)

TABLE 5–8
SKIN CANCER MUTATIONS[a]

Tumor	Mutation		
Dysplastic nevus, MM	p16/CDKN24		
SCC	P53		
SCC	↑$\alpha_6\beta_4$ integrin		
BCC	↓BP Ag2 → retraction artifact		
*BCC	Sonic Hedgehog (SHH)		
*BCC (BCNS)	Patched (PTC)		
		UV+	UV−
	PTC *wt*	–	–
	PTC (+/−)	BBC	–
	PTC (−/−)	BCC	BCC

[a] Smoothened (SMO) activates cell proliferation; normally, however, Patched (PTC), a transmembrane protein, inhibits SMO from doing so. If this inhibitory mechanism is removed either by a deficient or mutated PTC or by binding Sonic Hedgehog (SHH) to PTC, SMO signals cellular proliferation resulting in BCCs.

SUBTYPES OF SQUAMOUS CELL CARCINOMA

- Conventional
- Acantholytic/Adenoid
- Clear cell/mucin-producing
- Verrucous
- Spindle cell

SQUAMOUS CELL CARCINOMA: METASTATIC RATES

- Overall: 2%
- Sun-damaged skin: 0.5%
- Mucocutaneous: 11%
- Burn scar: 18%
- Chronic osteomyelitis: 31%
- Previous x-ray therapy: 20%
- SCC most common skin tumor that invades perineurally
- More likely to metastasize if there is perineural involvement
- Most common location of SCC in oral cavity: lateral tongue and floor of mouth
- UV-induced SCCs caused by change of CC nucleotides to TT
- Anogenital (HPV)

TYPES OF VERRUCOUS CARCINOMA

- Oral: oral florid papillomatosis
- Genital: Buschke-Lowenstein
- Plantar: epithelioma cuniculatum = rabbit burrow = amputation

CHAPTER

6

METABOLIC DISORDERS

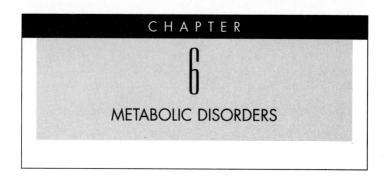

ACANTHOSIS NIGRICANS: TYPES

1. Benign: autosomal dominant
2. Obesity-associated: most common type
3. Syndromic:
   - Type A (HAIR-AN): hyperandrogenemia/insulin resistance—acanthosis nigricans
   - Type B: associated with connective tissue disease syndromes: scleroderma, Rud, Bloom, Lawrence-Seip, Crouzon
4. Malignant (oral mucosa, palms): gastric cancer, adenocarcinoma, bronchogenic carcinoma
5. Drug-induced: Niacin (cholesterol-lowering), oral contraceptives, steroids, diethylstilbestrol (DES)
6. Endocrine: hypo/hyperthyroidism, acromegaly

ACROMEGALY

- Hypertrophy of chin, nose, supraorbital ridges; drumstick fingers
- Thickened skin, not correlated with growth hormone level
- Cutis verticis gyrata in 30% of patients
- Treatment: bromocriptine, octreotide, or surgery

ADDISON DISEASE

- Darkening of mucous membranes, palmar creases, axillae, perineum, nipples, nevi
- Polyglandular syndrome: hypoparathyroidism, chronic candidal infection, vitiligo

TABLE 6–1
AMYLOID: TYPES

Type	Origin	Distribution/ Clinical Manifestations
SYSTEMIC		Mesenchymal (blood vessels, eccrine, fat)
Primary	AL-λ (bone marrow)	
Myeloma-associated	AL	Macroglossia, carpal tunnel, shoulder-pad sign, RA in small joints, purpura
Secondary	AA	
Familial Mediterranean	AA	Parenchymal organs (kidneys, liver, spleen)
Fever	AA	
Muckle-Wells syndrome	β-microglobulin	
Hemodialysis-associated	Transthyretin Prealbumin	Wrinkling of fingers, carpal tunnel syndrome
Familial amyloid	Gelsolin	
Neuropathy		
Senile cardiac myopathy		
Hereditary Finnish		
LOCALIZED		
Diabetes mellitus	Amylin	
Thyroid	Precalcitonin	
Hereditary cerebral	Cystatin C	
CUTANEOUS		
Primary		
Macular/lichenoid	Keratinocyte tonofilament	Papillary dermis Conchal + poikiloderma-like
Nodular	AL (local plasma cells)	Full thickness : F:M = 2:1, 60–70s, <15% progress to systemic disease; associated with Sjögren syndrome
Secondary		
BCC, Bowen's	Keratinocyte tonofilament	Adjacent tissue

Key: AL = amyloid light chain; AA = amyloid A protein.

TABLE 6–2
SYSTEMIC SECONDARY AMYLOID[a]

Arthritis	Infections	Chronic Cutaneous Disease	Other
Rheumatoid	Osteomyelitis	Stasis ulcer	Hodgkin
Psoriatic	Tuberculosis	Hidradenitis	Ulcerative colitis
	Leprosy	Dystrophic EB	
	Syphilis		
	Schistosomiasis		

[a] Diagnostic test is abdominal fat-pad biopsy: 95% are positive.

TABLE 6–3
DYSTROPHIC CALCIFICATION[a]

Connective Tissue	Genodermatoses	Other
Collagen vascular disease (dermatomyositis)	Ehlers-Danlos	Cutaneous tumor (pilomatricoma)
Panniculitis	Pseudo xanthoma elasticum (PXE)	Infection
Porphyria cutanea tarda (PCT)	Rothmund-Thompson	Trauma
Calciphylaxis, Raynaud's, esophageal dysmobility, sclerodactyly, telangiectasia (CREST)	Werner's	

[a] Result of local tissue injury or abnormalities.

TABLE 6–4
METASTATIC CALCIFICATION[a]

Chronic Renal Failure	↑Ca	Genodermatoses
Second-degree hyperparathyroidism	Hypervitaminosis D	Albright's hereditary osteodystrophy
Calciphylaxis	Milk-alkali syndrome	Pseudohyperparathy-roidism
	Sarcoidosis	

[a] Result of abnormal Ca/PO_4 metabolism.

IDIOPATHIC CALCIFICATION

- Tumoral calcinosis: familial disorder with high serum PO_4
- Iatrogenic: extravasation of calcium chloride, pentazocine, pitressin
- Treatment: warfarin (inhibit gamma-carboxy-glutamic acid), bisphosphonates, steroids, colchicine, aluminum hydroxide, diltiazem, probenecid, parathyroidectomy

CUSHING SYNDROME VS. DISEASE

- Central obesity, normal-appearing limbs, hypertrichosis, acne, high susceptibility to fungal infections, striae
- Syndrome secondary to adrenal tumor or exogenous cortisol; disease secondary to pituitary microadenoma (excess ACTH)
- Dexamethasone suppression test: 1mg given at 11 p.m., then check cortisol at 8 a.m.; > 10 μg/dL is diagnostic of Cushing disease

DIABETES-ASSOCIATED DISEASES

- Waxy skin + stiff joints
- Facial erythema (rubeosis facei)
- Xanthelasma
- Acanthosis nigricans
- Diabetic dermopathy
- Sclerederma of Buschker
- Generalized granuloma annulare (GA)
- Kyrle disease
- Bullous diabeticorum
- Cutaneous neuropathy (legs, sensory)
- Necrobiosis lipoidica diabeticorum (NLD)
- Clear cell syringoma

Reduced with Effective Control

- Staphyloccocal pyodermas
- Erythrasma
- Candidiasis
- Xanthomas
- Dermatophytosis

GOUT

- Primary: idiopathic elevation of uric acid levels
- Secondary: caused by thiazides, myeloproliferative disorders
- Fever occurs secondary IL-1 secretion after monosodium urate deposition
- Urine + pathology: needle-shaped crystals
- Treatment: uricosuric agents (probenicid), xanthine oxidase inhibitors (allopurinol)

TABLE 6–5
CLINICAL NUTRITIONAL DEFICIENCIES

Nutrient	Clinical Manifestations
Vitamin A	Phrynoderma "toad" skin (keratosis pilaris–like); night blindness + conjunctival Bitot spots (white), keratomalacia
Thiamine (vitamin B_1)	Red burning tongue, edema, cardiac enlargement
B_2 (riboflavin)	Oral-ocular-genital: cheilitis, photophobia, scrotal seborrhea
Niacin (vitamin B_3)	4Ds: diarrhea, dermatitis (Casal's necklace, scrotal erythema, seborrheic dermatitis), dementia, death (similar findings in tryptophan deficiency)
Vitamin B_6 (pyridoxine)	Atrophic glossitis with ulceration, seborrheic dermatitis, cheilitis
Vitamin B_{12} or folic acid	Glossitis, hyperpigmentation, canities
C (scurvy)	Perifollicular petechiae (hemorrhage), keratotic plugs, corkscrew hairs
Vitamin K	Purpura, hemorrhage, ecchymosis
Fe	Koilonychia, glossitis, cheilitis, telogen effluvium, dysphagia (Plummer-Vinson syndrome)
Biotin	Alopecia, lethargy, hypotonia, periorificial dermatitis, Brittle nails
Essential fatty acid	Occurs in TPN babies = periorificial dermatosis, lighter hair color, alopecia
Zinc	Acrodermatitis enteropathica (genetic or acquired) = Periorificial dermatitis; test: alkaline phosphatase or zinc
Selenium	Hypopigmentation
Copper	Light-colored, twisted hair
Protein-energy	Marasmus = prolonged deficiency, <60% ideal body weight (IBW), no edema Loss of buccal fat causes "monkey facies," dry, loose, wrinkled skin Kwashiorkor = protein deficiency, normal caloric intake, 60–80% IBW, edema Potbelly, "red" children, hypopigmented dry hair, "flaky paint" skin, "flag" sign of hair

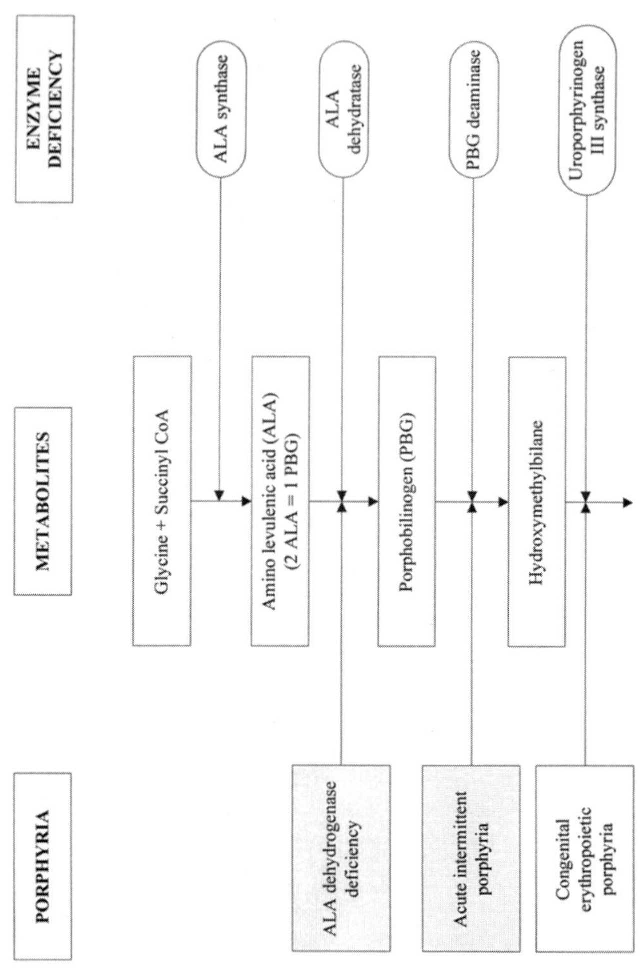

ENZYME DEFICIENCY
METABOLITES
PORPHYRIA
Glycine + Succinyl CoA
ALA synthase
Amino levulenic acid (ALA) (2 ALA = 1 PBG)
ALA dehydratase
Porphobilinogen (PBG)
PBG deaminase
Hydroxymethylbilane
Uroporphyrinogen III synthase
ALA dehydrogenase deficiency
Acute intermittent porphyria
Congenital erythropoietic porphyria

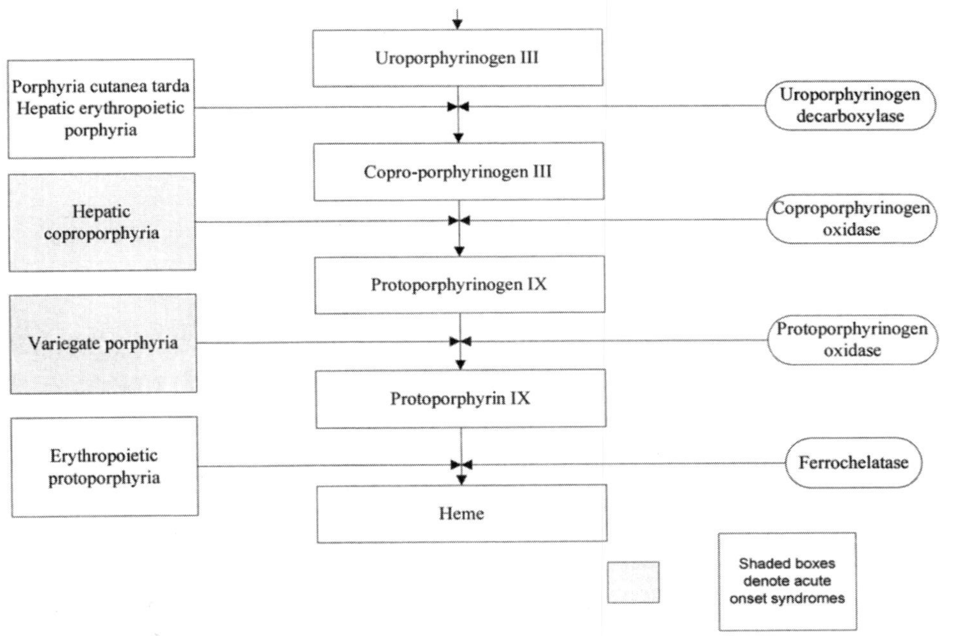

FIGURE 6–1
Porphyrin metabolic pathway.

PLUMMER-VINSON SYNDROME

- Microcytic anemia: glossitis, koilonychia
- Esophageal webs: dysphagia, cancer of mouth and upper respiratory tract

TABLE 6–6
PORPHYRIAS

Mnemonics: **A**ll **E**pstein **P**earls **H**ave **V**iolaceous **E**dges;
PUUC Proto Ferro DCDOO

Mnemonic	Type	Enzyme Deficiency		Location
All	**A**cute intermittent	**P**orphobilinogen	**D**eaminase	Cytosol
Epstein	**E**rythropoietic	**U**roporphyrinogen	**C**osynthase	Cytosol
Pearls	**PCT**	**U**roporphyrinogen	**D**ecarboxylase	Cytosol
Have	**H**ereditary coproporphyria	**C**oproporphyrinogen	**O**xidase	Mitochondria
Violaceous	**V**ariegate	**P**rotoporphyrinogen	**O**xidase	Mitochondria
Edges	**E**rythropoietic protoporphyria	**F**errochelatase		Mitochondria
HEP	Hepatoerythropoietic porphyria	Homozygous uroporphyrinogen decarboxylase		

TABLE 6–7
PORPHYRIA DIAGNOSTIC INDICATORS

Type[a]	Absorb	Emit	Urine	RBC	Stool	Flourescence
AIP	398 nm	619 nm	ALA, PBG	N	N	
EP	398 nm	619 nm	Uro (20 × Copro)	Uro	Copro	RBC (stable) and teeth
PCT	398 nm	619 nm	Uro (8 × Copro)	N	Isocopro	Urine (continuous)
HCP	398 nm	619 nm	Copro	N	Copro	
VP	405 nm	626 nm	Copro:Uro = 1:1 ALA,PBG	N	Proto	
EPP	409 nm	634 nm	N	Proto	Proto	RBC (transient)
HEP			Uro	Proto	Copro	
ECP			Copro	Copro	Copro	

[a] AIP = acute intermittent porphyria; EP = erythropoietic porphyria; PCT = porphyria cutanea tarda; HCP = hepatic coproporphyria; VP = variegate porphyria; EPP = erythropoietic protoporphyria; HEP = hepatic erythropoietic porphyria; ECP = erythropoietic coproporphyria.

- Watson-Schwartz test check for PBG.
- Delta-ALA synthetase = rate-limiting step located in mitochondria.
- Soret band = 400–410 nm.

TABLE 6–8
PORPHYRIAS: SPECIAL CLINICAL CHARACTERISTICS

Chronic erythropoietic porphyria (CEP)	Stained diaper Hyperbilirubinemia with blue light Blisters Need splenectomy
Erythropoietic protoporphyria (EPP)	Hypochromic microcytic anemia Cholelithiasis → liver failure → death Gallstones Need yellow filters on surgical lights to avoid phototoxic radiation 1. Fe deficiency 2. Pb poisoning
Erythropoietic coproporphyria (ECP)	Like EPP, but photosensitivity presents in infancy

PORPHYRIA AND ANTIMALARIALS

- Increase urinary uroporphyrin excretion
- Decrease hepatic porphyrin content
- No effect on delta-ALA-synthetase

PORPHYRIA (VARIEGATE)

Drug-induced. Mnemonic: **BEGS** for **ALCOHOL** or **SAFE**

Barbiturates
Estrogen
Griseofulvin
Sulfonamides
Alcohol

S = sulfas, sedatives, sex, steroids
A = anticonvulsants/alcohol
F = fungicides (griseofulvin linked to HCP)
E = ergots

PORPHYRIA WORKUP

1. Check hematocrit
2. Plasma porphyrin screen (wrap tube in foil)
3. 24-h urine in $NaCO_3$ buffered container; request quantitative Copro
4. 24-h stool

TABLE 6–9
XANTHOMAS

Lipid Δ[a]		Primary Cause	Secondary Cause–Associated	Xanthoma	Associations
I	↑↑Trig ↑chylo	Lipoprotein lipase deficiency (chylomicronemia I)		Eruptive	Lipemia retinalis, abd. pain, pancreatitis, hepatomegaly
IIA	↑LDL	↑Chol[[AU 13]] or familal hypercholestemia (FH) Apolipoprotein B defect (heterozygous)	Anorexia, porphyria hepatoma, nephrotic syndrome, porphyria myxedema,Cushing syndrome	Tendinous xanthelasma, tuberous xanthoma	CAD, CVAS
IIB	↑LDL ↑VLDL ↑Trig	FH Apolipoprotein B defect (homozygous)	Nephrotic syndrome, Cushing syndrome	Intertriginous tendinous xanthelasma	CAD, CVAs Advanced atherosclerosis
III	↑↑Trig ↑IDL	"Broad beta" disease Familial dysbetalipoproteinemia Apolipoprotein E defect	Paraproteinemia Obstructive liver disease	Palmar/plantar tendinous tuberous xanthoma	Diabetes, gout, obesity, CAD, CVAs
IV	↑↑Trig ↑VLDL	FH or Familial Hypertriglyceridemia	Diabetes, EtOH abuse Obesity, paraproteins	Eruptive tendinous/ tuberous xanthoma	CAD, CVAs, diabetes
V	↑↑Trig ↑chylo ↑VLDL	Type 5 hyperlipoproteinemia Apolipoprotein C2 defect (chylomicronemia II)	Diabetes, obesity, pancreatitis	Eruptive xanthoma	Hepatomegaly, lipemia retinalis, pancreatitis

[a] Tng = triglycerides; chylo = chylomicrons; Chol = cholesterol.

TABLE 6–10
DISORDERS AND XANTHOMA MORPHOLOGIES

	Cause	Defect	Characteristic Xanthoma
I	Chylomicronemia I	Lipoprotein lipase	Eruptive
IIA	Heterozygous FH	Apolipoprotein B	Tendinous
IIB	Homozygous FH	Apolipoprotein B	Intertriginous
III	Dysbetalipoproteinemia	Apolipoprotein E	Palmar
IV	Familial hypertriglyceridemia		Eruptive
V	Chylomicronemia II	Apolipoprotein C2	Eruptive

TABLE 6–11
CHARACTERISTIC LESION-SYNDROME ASSOCIATIONS

Xanthoma Type	Association
Intertirginous	Homozygous familial hypercholesterolemia (IIB)
Palmar	Familial dysbetalipoproteinemia (III)
	Obstructive liver disease (xanthomatous biliary cirrhosis)
Eruptive	Chylomicronemia (I + V)
Planar	Cholestasis
	Paraproteinemias
	Leukemia/lymphoma
Tendon	Heterozygous familial hypercholesterolemia (IIA)
	Cerebrotendinous xanthomatosis
	Phytosterolemia

CHAPTER

7

GENODERMATOSES

TABLE 7–1
ALBRIGHT HEREDITARY OSTEODYSTROPHY VS. McCUNE-ALBRIGHT SYNDROME

X-linked dominant	Autosomal dominant or sporadic
Osteodystrophy	Polyostotic fibrous dysplasia
Albright sign: dimpling of fifth metacarpal (not seen in pseudopseudohypoparathyroidism)	Endocrine dysfunction: precocious puberty (infantile vaginal bleeding)
Labs: pseudohypoparathryoidism (low PTH, high PO_4, low Ca) pseudopseudohypoparathyroidism (low PTH, normal PO_4, normal Ca)	Melanotic macule with ipsilateral bony changes

ALKAPTONURIA (OCHRONOSIS)

1. Defect: homogentisic acid oxidase deficiency (autosomal recessive)
2. Clinical: blue-gray pigment in skin, cartilage (destruction of ear), ligaments, tendon, sclera (Osler sign), dark diapers, brown sweat, arthropathy, intervetebral disk calcification
3. Pathology: yellow-brown swollen collagen bundles ("banana bodies"), dermis appears black with cresyl violet or methylene blue stain but negative with silver nitrate, iron, and lipofuscin stains.
4. Exogenous ochronsis: occurs after 6-month use of hydroquinone

MNEMONIC FOR DIFFERENTIAL DIAGNOSIS OF ANGIOID STREAKS

(Caused by breaks in Bruch membrane)
Apple pits:

Acromegaly
PXE
Paget disease of bone
Lead poisoning
Ehlers-Danlos syndrome
Pituitary/ ↑phosphate
Iron deficiency
Tuberous sclerosis/trauma
Sickle cell anemia
Cowden syndrome (13%)

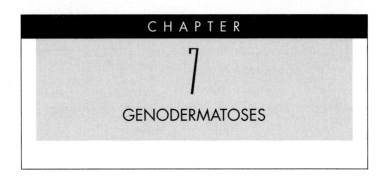

MNEMONIC FOR TYPES OF ANGIOKERATOMAS

Fabry circled the Ford around my Pappy:

Fabry	**F**abry disease	PAIN, Urine: Maltese crosses[a] and mulberry cells[b] (corpora diffusum)
Circled	**C**ircumscriptum	Congenital warty plaque
Ford	**F**ordyce	Scrotal (very common)
My	**M**ibelli	Dorsal digits, associated with chilblains
Pappy	**P**apular (solitary)	Lower extremities

[a] Maltese crosses: Lipid globules, seen with Oil Red O+ stain
[b] Mulberry cells: Glycosphingolipids in vascular endothelial cells creating lamellar structures on electron microscopy

DIFFERENTIAL DIAGNOSIS OF DIFFUSE ANGIOKERATOMAS

- α-Galactosidase A deficiency (Fabry disease)
- β-Galactosidase deficiency
- Fucosidosis
- Neuraminidase deficiency (sialidosis)
- β-Mannosidase deficiency
- Aspartylglycosaminase deficiency

ATOPIC DERMATITIS–ASSOCIATED SYNDROMES

- Wiskott-Aldrich disease
- X-linked hypogammaglobulinemia
- Chronic granulomatous disease
- Selective IgA deficiency
- Netherton syndrome
- Hartnup disease
- Histiocytosis X
- Ommen syndrome
- Ataxia-telangiectasia
- X-linked hyper-IgM syndrome
- Schwachman syndrome
- Phenylketonuria
- Anhidrotic ectodermal dysplasias
- Biotinylase deficiency
- Acrodermatitis enteropathica
- Arginosuccinic aciduria

TABLE 7–2
DIFFERENTIAL DIAGNOSIS OF CAFÉ-AU-LAIT (CAL) MACULES[a]

Syndrome	Prevalence	Clinical Features
SYNDROMES HAVING A *DEFINITE* ASSOCIATION WITH MULTIPLE OR SOLITARY CAL MACULES		
Neurofibromatosis 1	90%	Neurofibromas, iris hamartomas, osseous lesions, freckling, brain tumors, pheochromocytoma, neurofibrosarcoma, malignant schwannoma, Wilms tumor, "coast of California" CAL macules
Neurofibromatosis 2	60%	Eighth nerve masses, neurofibroma, meningioma, glioma, schwannoma, juvenile posterior subcapsular lenticular opacities
McCune-Albright syndrome	60%	Polyostotic fibrous dysplasia, precocious puberty (somatic mutation: G-protein), "coast of Maine" CAL macules
Ring chromosome syndrome	100%	Microcephaly, mental retardation, short stature, limb/cardiac abnormalities
Watson syndrome	90%	Pulmonic stenosis, freckling, low intelligence
SYNDROMES HAVING A *QUESTIONABLE* ASSOCIATION WITH CAL MACULES		
Bloom syndrome	0–50%	Photosensitivity, short stature, immunodeficiency, leukemia, lymphoma, GI malignancy, hypogonadism
Ataxia-telangiectasia	18–25%	Cerebellar ataxia, skin and eye telangiectasia, deficient thymus (↓IgA, G, E), lymphoma (T-cell type)
Tuberous sclerosis	15–30%	Seizures, mental retardation, facial angioma, hypomelanotic macules, CNS tumors
LEOPARD syndrome	38%	Lentigenes, pulmonic stenosis, hypertelorism, deafness
Silver-Russell syndrome	10–34%	Congenital short stature, limb asymmetry, triangular face

TABLE 7–2
DIFFERENTIAL DIAGNOSIS OF CAFÉ-AU-LAIT (CAL) MACULES (*Continued*)

Syndrome	Prevalence	Clinical Features
WHAT TO DO ABOUT CAL MACULES		
Solitary macule in white or black patient		No significance
If >3 in white patient		Follow up for development of multisystem disease
If >5 in white or black patient		Monitor closely for NF 1
If bone fractures or precocious puberty lines of hyperpigmentation (McCune-Albright)		Look for large macules or Blaschko

[a] The most common location for CAL macules in children: buttocks.

CALCIFICATION (INTRACRANIAL; GENODERMATOSES)

- Basal cell nevus syndrome (falx cerebri)
- Cockayne syndrome (brain)
- Sturge-Weber syndrome ("tram-track")
- Tuberous sclerosis (paraventricular = basal ganglia)
- Lipoid proteinosis hippocampus, ("bean-shaped" "sickle-shaped" sella turcica) (temporal lobe)
- Papillon-Lefevre (dural)

CANITIES (PREMATURE)

Syndromes		Autoimmune
Werner syndrome/ progeria	Ataxia-telangiectasia	Pernicious anemia
Fanconi syndrome	B_{12} (folate) deficiency	Thyroiditis
Rothmund-Thomson syndrome	Book syndrome	Vitiligo
Myotonia dystrophica	Seckel syndrome	Alopecia areata

DIFFERENTIAL DIAGNOSIS OF FOVEAL CHERRY-RED SPOTS

- Niemann-Pick disease
- Tay-Sachs disease
- Generalized sialidosis
- Sandhoff disease

DIFFERENTIAL DIAGNOSIS OF COLLODION BABY

- Normal
- Nonbullous congenital ichthyosiform erythroderma
- Lamellar ichthyosis
- Harlequin fetus
- Netherton syndrome (rarely)
- Chanarin-Dorfman neutral lipid storage disease (rarely)
- Gaucher disease type 2 (rarely)

COLONIC POLYPS—ASSOCIATED SYNDROMES

- Gardner
- Peutz-Jegher
- Familial polyposis coli
- Birt-Hogg-Dube
- Cronkhite-Canada
- Bannayan-Riley-Ruvalcaba

CONNECTIVE TISSUE NEVI: ASSOCIATED SYNDROMES

- Tuberous sclerosis (collagenoma = shagreen patch)
- Buschke-Ollendorf (elastoma, associated with osteopoikilosis)
- *Proteus* (collagenoma on plantar)
- MEN type 1

MNEMONIC FOR DOWN SYNDROME DERMATOSES

Cheaps:

C = cutis marmorata
H = hyperkeratosis/keratosis pilaris
E = elastosis perforans serpiginosa
A = elopecia areata
P = premature wrinkling
S = syringoma (20%)

TABLE 7–3
EHLERS-DANLOS SYNDROME

Type	Inheritance	Clinical	Defect
1: Gravis	AD	Lethal	Type 5 collagen
2: Mitis	AD	Less severe than gravis	Type 5 collagen
3: Benign	AD	Hypermobility (Gorlin's sign)	
4: Ecchymotic	AD	Aortic, GI, uterine rupture	Type 3 collagen synthesis
5: XL-R	XL-R		Lysyl oxidase error
6: Ocular	AR	Ocular fragility, marfanoid, retinal detachment, keratoconus	Lysyl hydroxylase deficency *PLOD* gene
7 A,B: Arthrochalasis	AD	Congenital hip dislocation	Type 1 procollagen defect
7 C: Dermatospraxis	AR	Very stretchable	Procollagen peptidase deficiency
8: Periodontal	AD	Periodontitis	
9: X-linked cutis laxa (occipital horn syndrome) (Menkes)	XL-R	Occipital exostosis, hernias, bladder rupture (Menkes kinky hair syndrome)	ATP7A gene: copper-binding ATPase Lysyl oxidase error
10: Fibronectin defect	AR	Easy bruising	Fibronectin[a]

[a] Repeats in fibronectin homologous to collagen VII, factor VIII, β4 integrin.

TABLE 7–4
ELASTIC FIBER DEFECTS

Disease	Defect	Pathology	Associations
Buschke-Ollendorf	↑ Desmosine	Thickened elastic fibers	Osteopoikilosis = long bones: coin-shaped opacities
Anetoderma	↓ Desmosine	Loss elastic fibers	
Cutis laxa	↓ Desmosine Cu-binding ATPase	Loss elastic fibers	Transient in baby associated with maternal penicillamine dosage
Menkes kinky hair	↓ Lysyl oxidase	Fragmented internal elastic lamina	
PXE	MRP6 gene	Fragmented + calcified elastic fibers	
Marfan syndrome	Fibrillin 1		Dissecting aorta (painless) Most common skin lesion is striae (60%) Spontaneous pneumothorax
Congenital contractural arachnodactyly	Fibrillin 2		

MNEMONIC FOR DIFFERENTIAL DIAGNOSIS OF ELASTOSIS PERFORANS SERPIGINOSA

Mad doper:

Marfan syndrome
Acrogyria
Down syndrome

D-penicillamine (causes "bramble-bush" pathologic appearance vs. "raveled-wool" in others)
Osteogenesis imperfecta
Pseudoxanthoma elasticum
Ehlers-Danlos syndrome
Rothmund-Thomson syndrome

Others: Scleroderma, XYY syndrome, renal disease

TABLE 7–5
EYE CHANGES IN GENODERMATOSES

Genodermatoses	Eye Changes
Basal cell nevus syndrome	Coloboma[a]
Goltz syndrome	Coloboma
Epidermal nevus syndrome	Coloboma, lipodermoids on conjunctiva = Schimmelpenning syndrome
Incontinentia pigmenti	Coloboma
X-linked ichthyosis	Corneal opacities: comma-shaped
Fabry syndrome	Corneal vertiselata = whorl-like opacities
Ehlers-Danlos syndrome	Angioid streaks, keratoconus,[b] ruptured globe, blue sclerae (type 6)
Atopic dermatitis	Keratoconus
Pachyonychia congenita III	Leukokeratosis of cornea
Nail-patella syndrome	Lester iris (hyperpigmentation of pupillary margin), heterochromic irides
Waardenburg syndrome	Heterochromic irides
Juvenile xanthogranuloma	Heterochromia irides, glaucoma, eye (iris) JXG lesions, hyphema
Down syndrome	Brushfield spots (iris)
Neurofibromatosis 1	Lisch nodules (iris)
Neurofibromatosis 2	Juvenile posterior subcapsular lenticular opacity/cataracts = 80%
Homocystinuria	Ectopia lentis: downward lens displacement
Marfan syndrome	Ectopia lentis: upward lens displacement
Wilson syndrome	Kayser-Fleischer rings
Von Hippel-Lindau syndrome	Retinal hemangioblastomas, leading to blindness
Tuberous sclerosis	Retinal phakomas, angioid streaks
Refsum syndrome	Retinitis pigmentosa: salt + pepper
Sjögren-Larsson syndrome	Retinitis pigmentosa: glistening dot
Cockayne syndrome	Retinitis pigmentosa: salt + pepper
Degos disease	Avascular patches on retina
Gardner syndrome	Congenital hypertrophied retinal pigmented epithelium (CHRPE)
Sturge-Weber syndrome	Glaucoma, ketchup-spot retina
Niemann-Pick disease	Cherry-red spots
Richner-Hanhart syndrome	Pseudoherpetic dendritic keratitis
Gaucher disease	Pingueculae[c]
Conradi-Hunnerman syndrome	Focal cataracts
PHACES syndrome	Cataracts
Rothmund-Thomson syndrome	50% cataracts by age 7
Werner syndrome	Cataracts
Hemangioma over eye	Amblyopia

[a] Coloboma = defect in embryogenic closure of optic stalk resulting in defect of any area of eye.
[b] Keratoconus = cone-shaped cornea.
[c] Pingueculae = elevation of tissue on conjunctiva lateral to cornea.

GAP JUNCTIONS

- Connexons—hexameric flower-like structures—that couple cells electrically and chemically
- Deficiency, which causes three things

  1. Vohwinkel syndrome with deafness = connexon 26
  2. Erythrokeratoderma variabilis = Connexon 31
  3. Hydrotic ectodermal dysplasia = possible connexon defect

OTHER GENETIC DEFECTS

- Plakophilin-1: mutation of both alleles → causes ectodermal dysplasia with skin fragility
- Desmoplakin haploinsufficiency causes striate palmoplantar keratoderma
- Desmoplakin-plakoglobin truncations cause striate palmoplantar keratoderma, woolly hair, and cardiomyopathy

HOMOCYSTINURIA

Defect: Cystathionine synthetase (methionine metabolism)
Clinical:

- MS: marfanoid (mental retardation not seen in Marfan syndrome)
- Skin: livedo reticularis, malar flush, DVTs
- Eye: downward lens dislocation
- Hair: fine, sparse

Labs: ↑ homocystine/ ↑ methionine in blood
Treatment: hydroxycobalamin, cyanocobalamin

HUNTER'S SYNDROME

- Inheritance: XL-R
- Defect: ↓ iduronate sulfatase/ ↑ dermatan and heparan sulfate
- Clinical: pebbling over scapula, coarse facies, short stature, hairy distal extremities

HYPERTRICHOSIS LANUGINOSA CONGENITA

- Associated with dental anomalies, gingival fibromatosis
- May be secondary to fetal hydantoin syndrome (characterized by depressed nasal bridge, large lips, short webbed neck)
- Other causes: fetal alcohol syndrome, minoxidil used during pregnancy

TABLE 7–6
ICHTHYOSIS SYNDROMES

Syndrome	Enzyme Deficiency	Clinical Manifestations
Refsum	Phytanoyl CoA α-hydroxylase	Retinitis pigmentosa (salt + pepper), ataxia
Rud		Hypogonadism, short stature
Sjögren-Larsson	Fatty aldehyde dehydrogenase	Spastic paresis, retinitis pigmentosa (glistening dot)
Trichothiodystrophy	↓ Cysteine (sulfur), XP-D defect	PIBIDS, trichoschisis, "tiger tail"
Netherton	SPINC-5	Ichthyosis linearis circumflexa, trichorrhexia invaginata, atopy
Conradi-Hünermann	Dihydroxy acetone phosphate acyltransferase (peroxisome) (DHAP)	Chondrodysplasia punctata, short limbs, whorled skin, stippled epiphyses
Chanarin-Dorfman	Neutral lipid storage disease	Lipid vacuoles in neutrophils, collodion baby
CHILD	Abnormal lamellar bodies ↓ peroxisomes	CHILD
KIDS		Keratitis ichthyosis, deafness, stippled palmoplantar keratoderma
Ichthyosis vulgaris	Profilaggrin/filaggrin/ keratohyalin	Flexures spared, hyperlinear palm
X-linked ichthyosis	Steroid sulfatase	Dirty, flexures/palms/ soles spared
Lamellar ichthyosis	Transglutaminase 1	Collodion baby, corrugated scale
Harlequin fetus	Odland bodies lacking	Collodion
Nonbullous congenital ichthyosiform erythroderma		Collodion, mild lamellar ichthyosis
Erythrokeratoderma variabilis	Connexin 31	Geographic changing keratotic plaques
Ichthyosis bullosa of Siemens	K2e	Mild epidermolytic hyperkeratosis-like features

TABLE 7–7
IMMUNODEFICIENCY SYNDROMES

Syndrome	Enzyme Deficiency	Clinical Manifestations
Wiskott-Aldrich	*WASP* (sialophorin = CD43) gene	Encapsulated bacteria, lymphoma, HSV, HPV
Severe combined immunodeficiency disorder (SCID)	IL-2Rγ (XLR), adenosine deaminase (AD)	Candidal infection
Leiner		Gram-negative bacteria
Chronic granulomatous disease	gp91 phos: cytochrome *b*-NADPH oxidase	Staph infection, nitro-blue tetrazolium test; carrier females susceptible to DLE and Jessner syndrome; treat with IFN-γ, which corrects enzyme dysfunction
Myeloperoxidase deficiency	Myeloperoxidase	Candidal infection
Chediak-Higashi	Giant lysosomes; *LYST* gene (chromosome 1q)	Staph infection, gray-silvery hair, malignant lymphoma
Hyper IgD		Periodic fever, diarrhea, joints; triggers: vaccines, viruses, stress
Hyper IgE = Job syndrome		Sterile pyoderma, eczema
Hyper IgM	gp39	Oral ulcerations
Hypereosinophilia	IL-5 (Th2) overexpression	Oral ulcerations, angioedema; treated with steroids
X-linked agammaglobulinemia	↓B cells	Bacterial; echovirus induces dermatomyositis-like syndrome
X-linked lymphoproliferative syndrome		Viral, EBV
Leukocyte adhesion deficiency type 1 (LAD-1)	β_2-integrin deficiency	Delayed umbilical cord separation

LENS DISPLACEMENT

- Upward ↑ displacement associated with Marfan syndrome
- Downward ↓ displacement associated with homocystinuria

LEOPARD SYNDROME

Mnemonic: LEOPARD

Lentigenes
ECG changes
Ocular hypertelorism
Pulmonic stenosis
Abnormal genitals
Retarded growth
Deafness

LYSYL OXIDASE DEFICIENCY

- Ehlers-Danlos syndrome type IX
- Cutis laxa
- Menkes kinky hair syndrome
- Vitamin C deficiency

TABLE 7–8
TYPES OF MULTIPLE ENDOCRINE NEOPLASIA (MEN)

MEN Type I	MEN Type IIA	MEN Type IIB (Sipple Syndrome)
Chromosome 11: menin automosal dominant	Thyroid medullary carcinoma: check calcitonin	Thyroid medullary carcinoma
Parathyroid gland cancer; adenomas most common	Pheochromocytoma (50%): check urine catecholamines	Pheochromocytomas
Pancreatic cancer: insulinomas (21%) glucagonomas (13%) = necrolytic migratory erythema	Elevated parathyroid hormone (10%)	Mucosal neuromas ("blubbery lips")
	Lichen amyloidosis (or macular)	Marfanoid habitus
	Usually interscapular	CAL macules
		GI ganglioneuromatosis = megacolon
Pituitary: anterior carcinoma	*ret* protooncogene (extra-cellular domain defect-receptor)	
Gastric: gastrinomas (54%)		
Thyroid: follicular adenoma		*ret* protooncogene (intracellular domain defect-protein kinase)
Adrenal gland: adenomas		
Foregut: carcinoid tumor		
Angiofibromas (facial)		
Connective tissue nevi		
CAL and confetti macules		
Lipomas, gingival papules		

MONILETHRIX

Defect: keratins 1, 6
Hair: beaded with undulating diameter
Associated with:

- Keratosis pilaris (K6 mutation), tooth abnormalities
- Rarely—cataracts, mental retardation

MUCKLE-WELLS SYNDROME

- Amyloidosis
- Urticaria
- Deafness
- Fever and parasthesias

NAME SYNDROME (CARNEY COMPLEX)

Mnemonic: NAME

Nevi
Atrial myxoma
Myxoid neurofibromas (psammomatous melanotic schwannoma)
Ephelides

Also two or more of the following:

- Cardiac myxomas (79%)
- Cutaneous myxomas (45%)
- Mammary myxoid fibromas (30%)
- Spotty pigmentation (65%)
- Pigmented nodular adrenocortical disease (45%)
- Testicular tumors (56%)
- Pituitary growth hormone tumors (10%)

TABLE 7–9
NEUROCUTANEOUS SYNDROMES → GENETIC DEFECTS[a]

Syndrome	Defect	Chromosome
Neurofibromatosis 1	Neurofibromin → GAPs (-) protooncogene *p21-ras*	17
Neurofibromatosis 2	Merlin → tumor suppressor (associated with meningioma)	22
Tuberous sclerosis	Tuberin (TS-2, chromosome 16) → GTPase activating protein rap 1 (tumor suppressor gene)	9, 16
	Hamartin (TS-1, chromosome 9)	4
Piebaldism	c-*kit* protooncogene (mast cell growth factor receptor)	

[a] Neurocutaneous melanosis: giant congenital nevus (bathing trunk), increased intracranial pressure, photophobia, possible tethered cord.

DIAGNOSTIC CRITERIA FOR NEUROFIBROMATOSIS 1

Two or more of the following:

$\geqslant$6 CAL macules $\geqslant$0.5 cm (prepubertal) or $\geqslant$1.5 cm (postpubertal)
$\geqslant$2 NFs of any type or 1 plexiform NF
Freckling in axilla or groin (Crowe sign)
Optic glioma; brain tumors
$\geqslant$2 Lisch nodules
Bony lesions/abnormalities (pseudoarthrosis, sphenoid wing dysplasia causes pulsating exophthalmos, scoliosis most common)
First-degree relative with NF-1

TABLE 7–10
ORDER OF APPEARANCE OF LESIONS

Café-au-lait (CAL) macules	90% at 1 year
Axillary freckling	90% at 7 years
Lisch nodules	70% at 10 years
Neurofibromas	50% at 10 years and 84% at 20 years

DEFECTS IN OCULOCUTANEOUS ALBINISM (OCA)

- OCA-1 = tyrosinase
- OCA-2 = *P* gene: most common in African Americans
- OCA-3 = tyrosinase-related protein 1 (TRP-1)

TABLE 7–11
PALMOPLANTAR KERATODERMAS (PPKs)

Disease	Defect	Clinical Manifestations
Vohwinkel syndrome	Loricrin, GJB2 (connexin 31)	Honeycomb PPK, starfish keratoses, pseudoainhum, deaf
Unna-Thost	K1	Knuckle pads, hyperhidrosis
Howel-Evans syndrome	↓Envoplakin	Esophageal cancer, thick yellow palms and soles
Olmsted syndrome		Periorificial, ainhum
Mal de Meleda		Transgrediens, koilonychia, onychogryphosis, intertriginous psoriasiform plaques
Papillon-Lefevre syndrome		Transgrediens, periodontitis, dural cancer
Hidrotic ectodermal dysplasia		Transgrediens PPK
Richner-Hanhart syndrome	Tyrosine amino-transferase	Painful keratitis
Vorner syndrome	K9	Knuckle pads, epidermolytic
KIDS syndrome		Stippled PPK
Pachydermoperiostosis		Windblown desert, rippled PPK

MNEMONIC: PHACES

Posterior fossa Dandy-Walker abnormalities (also may be caused by neurocutaneous melanosis)
Hemangioma (large on face)
Arterial anomalies
Cardiac anomalies, including coarctation of the aorta
Eye abnormalities (cataracts)
Sternum abnormalities (clefting, supraumbilical raphe)

PILI TORTI

Defect unknown
Hair: twisted 180 degrees
Differential diagnosis: with deafness, Bjornstad syndrome; with hypogonadism, Crandall syndrome

- Menkes kinky hair syndrome
- Bazex syndrome
- Isotretinoin/acitretin therapy
- Corkscrew hair syndrome
- Trichothiodystrophy
- Rapp-Hodgkin hypohidrotic ectodermal dyplasia
- Citrullinemia (arginosuccinate synthetase deficiency)

MNEMONIC: POEMS SYNDROME

Associated with glomeruloid hemangioma (Crow-Fukase syndrome)

Polyneuropathy
Organomegaly
Endocrinopathy
M protein (IgG paraproteinemia)
Skin lesions: ↑pigment, edema, ↑sweating, hypertrichosis, thickening, clubbed nails, leukonychia, angiomas (glomeruloid), sclerodermoid features [associated with Castleman disease (HHV-8)]

TABLE 7–12
SEVERE COMBINED IMMUNODEFICIENCY DISORDER (SCID)

	Autosomal Dominant		X-Linked Recessive
Defect	Adenosine deaminase deficiency		Gamma (γ)-chain of IL-2 receptor
Clinical	**S**	**S**eborrheic dermatitis	
	C	**C**andidal infections	
	I	**I**L-2 receptor (γ-chain) defect (XL-R)	
	D	**D**eficient thymus	

↑ SISTER CHROMATID EXCHANGE

Mnemonic: Baby chromatids die frequently.

B = **B**loom syndrome
C = **C**ockayne syndrome
D = **D**yskeratosis congenita
F = **F**anconi syndrome

[Ataxia-telangiectasia has increased chromosomal breaks (not sister exchange).]

TABLE 7–13
SPHINGOLIPIDOSES

Disease	Enzyme Deficiency	Clinical Manifestations	Electromicroscopy
Niemann-Pick disease	Sphingomyelinase	Waxy indurated skin, mental retardation	Myelin bodies
Gaucher disease	Glucocerebrosidase	Pingueculae	
Fabry syndrome	α-Galactosidase A	Angiokeratomas	Lamellar inclusions
Fucosidosis	α-L-Fucosidase	Angiokeratomas	
Sialidosis	Neuraminidase	Angiokeratomas	
Farber disease (lipogranulomatosis)	Ceramidase	Hoarseness, periarticular nodules	Curvilinear, zebra bodies, banana bodies

STURGE-WEBER SYNDROME

- V1 unilateral = 10% with Sturge-Weber
- V1 bilateral = 40% with Sturge-Weber
- Homolateral leptomeningeal angiomatosis leads to epilepsy, hemiplegia
- Ocular involvement: glaucoma, retinal detachment, blindness (50% patients)

TRICHORRHEXIS NODOSA

Defect: arginosuccinase deficiency
Hair: interlocking brooms
Differential diagnosis:

- Arginosuccinic aciduria
- Citrullinemia
- Menkes kinky hair
- Netherton syndrome

TRICHOTHIODYSTROPHY

- Defect: ↓ sulfur/cystine content; *XP-D* gene defect = defect in repair of UVB-induced DNA damage
- Hair: tiger tail (polarizing light microscopy), trichoschisis = hair shaft breakage, ↓ cystine in hair
- Clinical: mnemonic—PIBIDS

  Photosensitivity
  Ichthyosis
  Brittle hair
  Intellectual impairment
  Decreased fertility
  Short stature

TABLE 7–14
X-RAY (AND CT/MRI) FINDINGS IN GENODERMATOSES

Finding	Syndrome/Disorder
Osteopathia striata	Goltz
Osteopoikilosis	Buschke-Ollendorf
Polyostotic fibrous dysplasia	McCune-Albright
Osteodystrophy	Albright
Chrondrodysplasia punctata	Conradi-Hünermann (occasionally CHILD)
Dyschondroplasia	Maffucci
Tufted phalanges	Hidrotic ectodermal dysplasia
Achondroplasia	Cartilage-hair hypoplasia
Metaphyseal widening + long bone spurs	Menkes kinky hair
Radial head subluxation	Nail-patella
Posterior iliac horns	
Thick scapulae	
Intervertebral disk calification (severe arthropathy)	Alkaptonuria
Ehrlenmeyer flask deformity of femur	Gaucher
Absent thymus on chest x-ray	SCID, DiGeorge, and Nezeloff
Osteoporosis	Reflex sympathetic dystrophy
Exostosis, macrodactyly, and scoliosis	*Proteus*
Distal phalangeal radiolucency	Incontinentia pigmenti → painful subungual verrucous lesions

UNCOMBABLE HAIR SYNDROME

Defect unknown

Hair: triangular configuration of hair shaft, longitudinal groove on electron microscopy

Synonyms:

- Cheveux incoiffables
- Spun-glass hair
- Pili triangulati et canaliculi

VON HIPPEL–LINDAU SYNDROME

- Retinal hemangioblastoma
- Renal cell cancer
- Pheochromocytoma
- VHL gene = tumor suppressor gene

WISKOTT-ALDRICH SYNDROME (WAS)

Mnemonic: Texas

Thrombocytopenia
Eczema
X-linked recessive
A: ↑IgA, ↑IgD, ↑IgE
Sialophorin

a. Inheritance: XL-R
b. Defect: CD43 "sialophorin" glycoprotein on leukocytes and platelets
c. Gene: WASP (WAS protein) → lymphocyte signal transduction
d. Clinical:
    - Eczema/eczema herpeticum (HSV)
    - Pyogenic infections (encapsulated organisms)
    - Purpura, bloody diarrhea, epistaxis
    - 10% with lymphoma/leukemia at a young age
e. Ig profile
    - ↓ IgM, IgG
    - ↑ IgA, IgD, IgE

TABLE 7–15
XERODERMA PIGMENTOSUM

Type	Defect	Clinical Manifestations
A	Recognize UV-damaged DNA	DeSanctis-Cacchione; Japan, dwarf, choreathetosis, mental retardation, ataxia, deafness
B	DNA helicase (Cockayne)	Dwarf, increased melanoma = Cockayne
C	Global genome repair	Only cutaneous findings. Most common xeroderma pigmentosum found in USA
D	Helicase	Defect also causes trichothiodystrophy
G	Endonuclease	Neurologic only

X-LINKED DOMINANT DISORDERS

Mnemonic: AGICCO

Albright hereditary osteodystrophy (variant)/Aicardie syndrome (colobomas)
Goltz
Incontinentia pigmenti
CHILD syndrome
Conradi-Hünermann syndrome
Oral-digital-facial syndrome

X-LINKED AGAMMAGLOBULINEMIA

(Bruton hypogammaglobulinemia)

- Rheumatoid arthritis-like
- Dermatomyositis-like eruption after echovirus infection

X-LINKED LYMPHOPROLIFERATIVE DISEASE

(Duncan disease)

- Inadequate response to EBV infection
- Life-threatening mononucleosis
- → Lymphoma

X-LINKED RECESSIVE DISORDERS

Mnemonic: Chad's kinky wife (and other stuff)

Chronic granulomatous disease
Hunter syndrome
Anhidrotic ectodermal dysplasia
Dyskeratosis congenita
SCID
Menkes **K**inky hair
Wiskott-Aldrich syndrome
Ichthyosis X-linked
Fabry syndrome
Ehlers-Danlos (types 5 and 9 syndrome

Other stuff

- Hyper-IgM syndrome
- X-linked agammaglobulinemia (Bruton syndrome)
- X-linked lymphoproliferative disease (Duncan syndrome)
- Keratosis follicularis spinulosa Decalvans
- Crandall syndrome (variant of Bjornstad syndrome and pili torti)
- Lesch-Nyhan syndrome

TABLE 7–16
X-RAY (AND CT/MRI) FINDINGS IN GENODERMATOSES

Finding	Syndrome/Disorder
Osteopathia striata	Goltz
Osteopoikilosis	Buschke-Ollendorf
Polyostotic fibrous dysplasia	McCune-Albright
Osteodystrophy	Albright
Chrondrodysplasia punctata	Conradi-Hunnerman (occasionally CHILD)
Dyschondroplasia	Maffucci
Tufted phalanges	Hidrotic ectodermal dysplasia
Achondroplasia	Cartilage-hair hypoplasia
Metaphyseal widening + long bone spurs	Menkes kinky hair
Absent patella	Nail-patella
Radial head subluxation	
Posterior iliac Horns, bilateral thick scapulae	
Intervertebral disk calification (severe arthropathy)	Alkaptonuria
Ehrlenmeyer flask deformity of femur	Gaucher
Absent thymus on chest x-ray	SCID, DiGeorge, Nezelof syndromes
Osteoporosis	Reflex sympathetic dystrophy
Exostosis and scoliosis	*Proteus* syndrome
Distal phalangeal radiolucency	Incontinentia pigmenti → painful subungual verrucous lesions
Absent radius	Rothmund-Thomson
Periostosis of long bones	Pachydermoperiostosis
Scoliosis	Ichthyosis hystrix, neurofibromatosis 1
Tram-track calcifications on head CT	Sturge-Weber
Odontogenic cysts in jaw	Basal cell nevus
Enchondromas	Mafucci (sarcomatous degeneration occurs in 50% of patients)
Sphenoid wing dysplasia	Neurofibromatosis 1
Stippled epiphyses	Conradi-Hünermann

CHAPTER

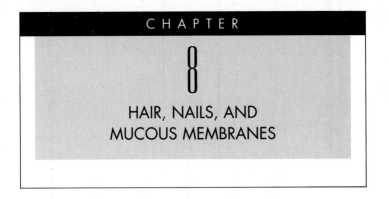

HAIR, NAILS, AND MUCOUS MEMBRANES

APOCRINE GLANDS

- Axillae, anogenital, external ear canal (ceruminous glands), eyelids (Moll's glands), breast (mammary)
- Active in puberty
- Chromhidrosis secondary to lipofuscin

APPENDAGEAL STRUCTURES (EMBRYOGENESIS)

Occurs between 18 and 24 weeks' gestation.
Mnemonic: Have sex every afternoon.

Hair
Sebaceous
Eccrine
Apocrine

CHEILITIS

- Glandularis: lower lip.
- Volkmann: suppurative type leads to permanent swelling; May also lead to SCC.
- Granulomatosa: upper lip.
- Angular: infectious (candidal or bacterial), mechanical (malocclusion or edentulousness), nutritional deficiency (riboflavin, folate, iron).
- Contact: primary irritant due to lip-licking, especially in atopic dermatitis; secondary irritant contact by extension from surrounding skin due to lipsticks (azo dyes, lanolin, perfumes), mouthwash (mint oils), toothpastes (fluoride, cinnamon), food (oranges, mangoes, artichokes).
- Actinic: high potential for SCC.

ECCRINE GLANDS

Innervated by sympathetic cholinergic (acetylcholinergic) fibers.
Absent in:

- Nail bed
- Vermilion border
- Glans penis and prepuce
- Labia

TABLE 8–1
HAIR ABNORMALITIES/DISEASES

Abnormality	Microscopic Appearance	Diseases
Telogen	Rounded bulb, no sheath	Telogen effluvium
Anagen	distorted bulb, sheath, tapered ends	Anagen effluvium, normal
"Exclamation point"	Attenuated "exclamation point" bulb	Alopecia areata
Trichorrhexis nodosa	"Double broomstick"	Argininosuccinicaciduria, Menkes kinky hair, Netherton syndrome, citrullinemia, hypothyroidism; weakest tensile strength
Trichorrhexis invaginata	"Ball-in socket"	Netherton syndrome (ichthyosis linearis circumflexa)
Pili torti	"Twisted hair"	Bjornstad, Menkes kinky hair, Crandall syndromes
Beaded hair	Narrowing = beads = weakest point	Monilethrix
Pili tranguli et canaliculi	"triangular shaft," long groove on EM	Uncombable hair syndrome
Pili multigemini	Bifurcated matrices/papillae	Cleidocraniodysostosis
Trichostasis spinulosa	Nose, back, tuft vellus hair, telogen hair retention	Treat with keratolytics
Trichoschisis	"Tiger tail"	Trichothiodystrophy (PIBIDS)
Coiled hairs	Screw-like configuration	Woolly hair syndrome
"Baggy sock"	Ruffled cuticle wrapped around hair	Loose anagen hair syndrome (98–100% anagen hairs, resolves with time)

“Bubble”	Bubbles in shaft	Blow-dryer hair
Pili annulati	Ringed pigment bands	Normal tensile strength, normal growth; strongest
Pohl Pinkus	Beau lines in hair	Hair loss after chemotherapy (anagen effluvium)
Longitudinal groove (EM)		Uncombable hair, anhidrotic ectodermal dysplasia
Light-colored hair		PKU secondary to low tyrosine
Bleached hair		Homocystinuria
Silvery hair		Griscelli syndrome, Chediak-Higashi syndrome
Red-blond hair		Kwashiorkor
White roots		Chloroquine
Canities		Vitamin B_{12} deficiency, interferon
Green hair		Copper; treat with chelating shampoo (penicillamine shampoo)

Note: Cytochrome P450 aromatase in frontal hair follicles protects against androgenetic alopecia.

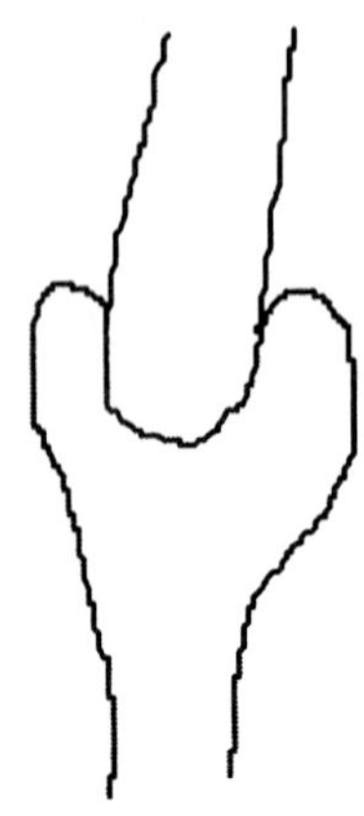

Trichorrhexis invaginata

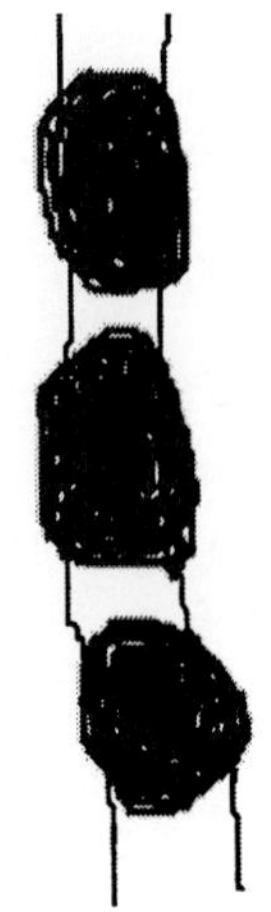

Monilethrix

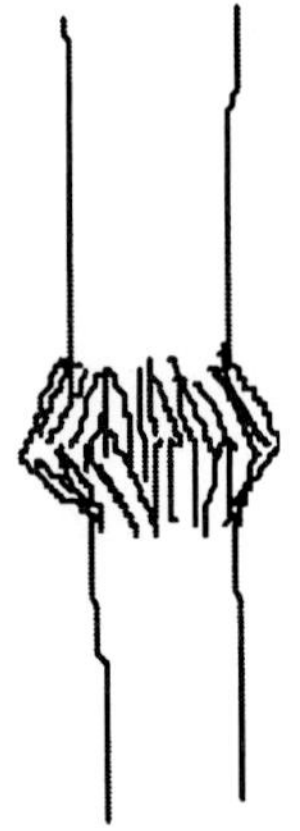

Trichorrhexis nodosa

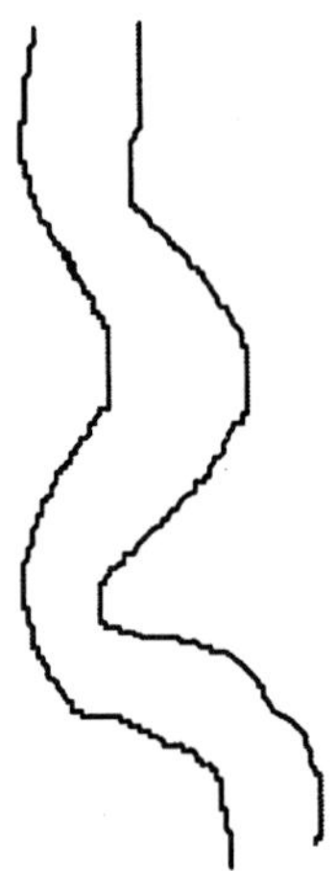

Pili torti

FIGURE 8–1
Abnormalities of the hair shaft.

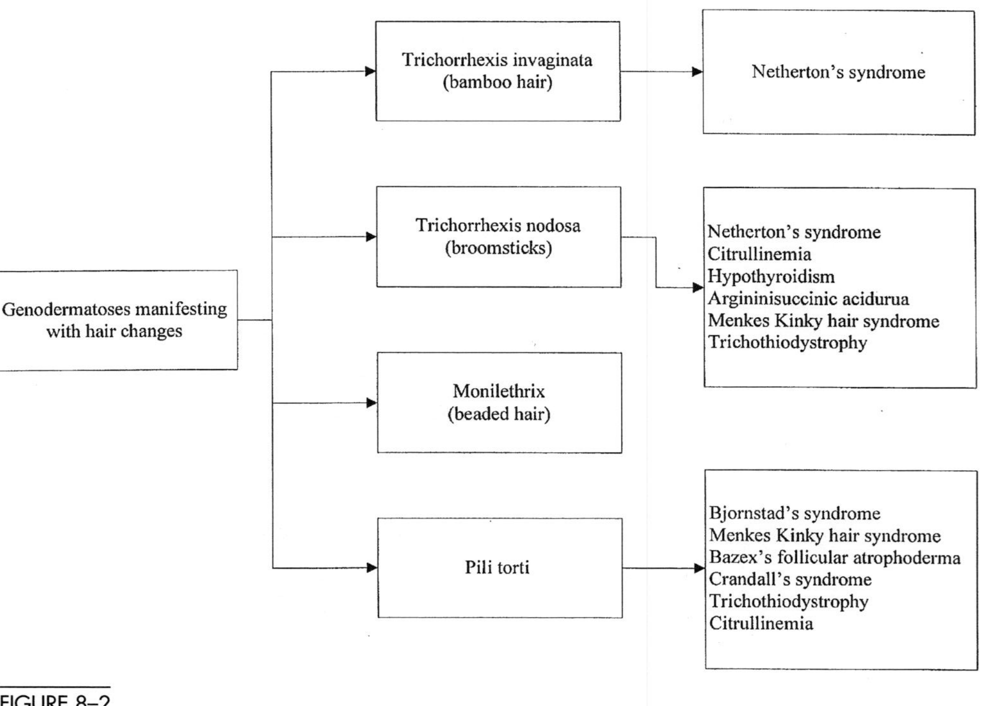

FIGURE 8–2
Genodermatoses and abnormalities of the hair shaft.

HAIR CASTS

- Occurs in females secondary to traction
- White keratinous sleeve slides easily
- Blue-yellow fluorescence with Wood's lamp

TABLE 8–2
HAIR CYCLE

Anagen	3 years, 84% scalp hair
Telogen	3 months, 14% scalp hair
Catagen	3 weeks, 2% scalp hair

HAIR GROWTH

- Normal: 0.35 mm/day
- After hair transplantion: 3–6 months

TABLE 8–3
HAIR STRUCTURE (CONTENT)

Structure	Content	Location
Infundibulum		Epidermis
Dermal papillae	Embryonic mesenchyme	
Isthmus	Trichilemmal keratinization (no trichohyalin)	Dermis
Inner root sheath	Trichohyalin, citrulline	
Medulla	Trichohyalin, citrulline	
Bulb		Subcutis

Note: Follicular units each have 1–3 hairs; Bulb and bulge contain melanocytes.

ORDER OF HAIR KERATINIZATION

1. Henle layer
2. Cuticle
3. Huxley layer

TABLE 8–4
HAIR SHAFT AND INNER ROOT SHEATH

←←←INNER TO OUTER→→→

Hair Shaft			Inner Root Sheath			Outer Root Sheath
Medulla	Cortex	Cuticle	Cuticle	Huxley[a]	Henley[b]	

[a] Mnemonic: Huxley hugs the cuticle.
[b] Mnemonic: Hens are outside in the outhouse.

HIRSUTISM

Hair growth limited to androgen

- sensitive areas

HYPERTRICHOSIS

Hair growth not limited to androgen-sensitive areas

DIFFERENTIAL DIAGNOSIS OF HIRSUTISM

- Polycystic ovaries (80%)
- Hyperandrogenism, insulin resistance, and acanthosis nigricans (HAIR-AN) syndrome
- Congenital adrenal hyperplasia (including late hereditary)
- Androgenic tumors
- Prolactinoma
- Cushing disease
- Idiopathic

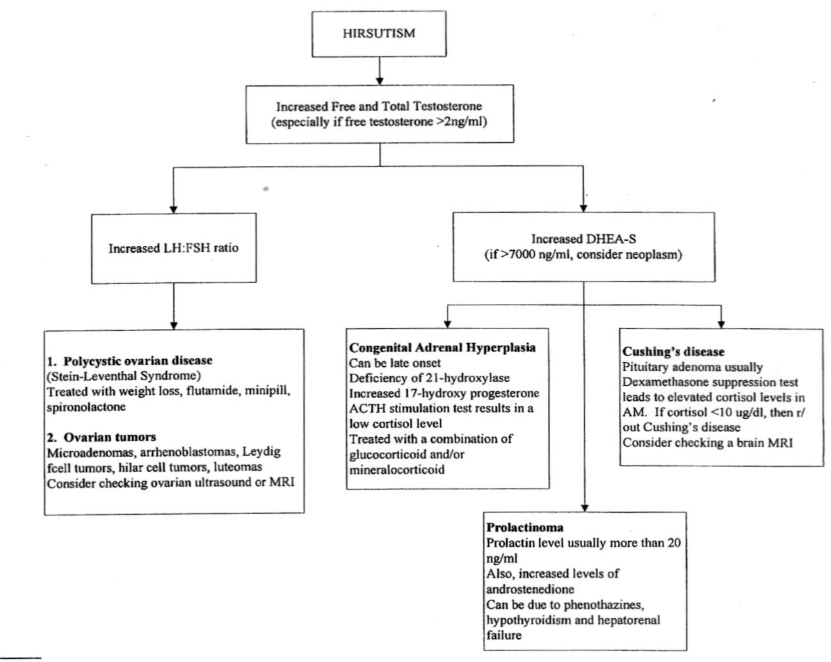

HIRSUTISM
Increased Free and Total Testosterone
(especially if free testosterone >2ng/ml)
Increased LH:FSH ratio
Increased DHEA-S
(if >7000 ng/ml, consider neoplasm)
1. Polycystic ovarian disease
(Stein-Leventhal Syndrome)
Treated with weight loss, flutamide, minipill, spironolactone
2. Ovarian tumors
Microadenomas, arrhenoblastomas, Leydig fcell tumors, hilar cell tumors, luteomas
Consider checking ovarian ultrasound or MRI
Congenital Adrenal Hyperplasia
Can be late onset
Deficiency of 21-hydroxylase
Increased 17-hydroxy progesterone
ACTH stimulation test results in a low cortisol level
Treated with a combination of glucocorticoid and/or mineralocorticoid
Cushing's disease
Pituitary adenoma usually
Dexamethasone suppression test leads to elevated cortisol levels in AM. If cortisol <10 ug/dl, then r/out Cushing's disease
Consider checking a brain MRI
Prolactinoma
Prolactin level usually more than 20 ng/ml
Also, increased levels of androstenedione
Can be due to phenothazines, hypothyroidism and hepatorenal failure

FIGURE 8–3
Workup and treatment of hirsutism.

TABLE 8–5
SYNOPSOIS OF SYNDROMES ASSOCIATED WITH HIRSUTISM

Disease	Etiopathogenesis	Treatment
Polycystic ovarian disease (PCOD)	Ovarian cysts result in ↑LH:FSH ratio	Weight loss, flutamide, minipill (progesterone), aldactone, cyproterone
Congenital adrenal hyperplasia (CAH)(late)	Deficiency of 21-hydroxylase, 11β-hydroxylase, or 3β-(OH) steroid dehydrogenase results in ↑17(OH) progesterone; ACTH stimulation test shows ↓cortisol	Flucortisone (mineralocorticoid + glucocorticoid), dexamethasone

TREATMENT OF HIRSUTISM

Leuprolide: GnRH agonist for precocious puberty and hirsute women
Finasteride: inhibitor of 5α-reductase type 2
DHT most potent androgen
Spironolactone: inhibits

- 17α-monooxygenase
- Androgen synthesis
- Androgen receptor
- 5α-reductase

HYPERHIDROSIS

Congenital	Vascular
PPK (Unna-Thost) Pachyonychia congenital Ichthyosis Nevus sudoriferous (eccrine nevus)	Glomus tumor Blue-rubber-bleb nevus
Generalized	**Other**
Psoriasis Infectious: malaria, tuberculosis Lymphoma Endocrine: diabetes, hyperthyroid, hyperpituitarism, pheochromocytoma Cold sweats: drugs, shock, hypoglycemia Carcinoid	Apocrine chromhidrosis caused by lipofuscin Compensatory, caused by sympathectomy Reflex sympathetic dystrophy
Gustatory	
Pancoast tumor Diabetes Postzoster complications Parotitis Frey auriculotemporal syndrome after parotid surgery	

LEUKOPLAKIA

- Premalignant change or may be due to smoking, malocclusion, ill-fitting dentures.
- Does not wipe off, like *Candida*.
- Pediatric premalignant leukoplakia is associated with dyskeratosis congenita.

DIFFERENTIAL DIAGNOSIS OF BLUE LUNULA

- Argyria
- AZT (zidovudine)
- Wilson disease
- Phenolphthalein
- Chemotherapy
- Hemoglobin M

DIFFERENTIAL DIAGNOSIS OF RED LUNULA

- Alopecia areata
- CO poisoning
- Psoriasis/rheumatoid arthritis
- Cardiovascular disease
- Lichen sclerosus
- Vitiligo
- COPD
- Collagen vascular disease with prednisone
- Lichen planus

NAIL FACTOIDS

- Little melanin, hence little photoprotection in the nail bed.
- Lack of stratum granulosum.
- No sebaceous glands.
- UVA penetrates normal nails more readily than it penetrates normal skin.

CAUSES OF ABSENT NAILS

- Epidermolysis bullosa syndromes
- Lamellar ichthyosis
- Dyskeratosis congenita
- Nail-patella syndrome
- KID syndrome
- Rothmund-Thomson syndrome
- Hidrotic ectodermal dysplasia
- Trisomy 8

CAUSES OF BLUE NAILS—SECONDARY TO DISEASE

- Hemochromatosis
- Wilson disease
- Ochronosis/alkaptonuria

CAUSES OF YELLOW NAILS

Secondary to lipofuscin

- Bronchiectasis
- Lymphedema/Milroy disease
- Rheumatoid arthritis
- Thyroid disease
- COPD
- Malignancies (breast, gallbladder, CTCL)
- D-penicillamine
- Chronic sinusitis/bronchitis
- Lichen planus (toenails only)
- Idiopathic pleural effusions
- Chronic sinusitis
- Immunodeficiencies (AIDS)

TABLE 8–6
SYSTEMIC DISEASES AFFECTING THE NAILS[a]

Type	Clinical Manifestations	Systemic Disease
Muehrcke	Paired horizontal white bands (nail bed)	Hypoalbuminemia secondary to nephrotic syndrome
Terry	Proximal 2/3 white, distal 1/3 red	Hypoalbuminemia secondary to cirrhosis or CHF
Half + half (Lindsay)	Proximal 1/2 white, distal 1/2 pink	CRF
Mees lines	Horizontal leukonychia, defect nail plate	Arsenic poisoning
Beau lines	Apical matrix arrest	Physiologic insult
Koilonychia	Spoon-shaped, concave nails	Iron deficiency, mal de Meleda, hyperthyroid, etc.
Trachyonychia	20-nail dystrophy	Alopecia areata
Onychoschizia	Splitting	Lichen planus
Pterygium unguium inversum	Inverse pterygium starting from hyponychium	Scleroderma, trauma, reaction to formaldehyde-containing nail polish
Oncyhorrhexis	Brittle nails	Hypothyroidism, retinoids, thalidomide; treat with biotin
Onycholysis	Yellow discolorations of plate; defect of distal lunular (ventral) matrix	Hyperthyroidism, tetracycline (photoonycholysis), 8-MOP, mercaptopurine (photo), quinolones, chloramphenicol
Onychomadesis	Periodic total nail shedding; separation at proximal nail fold	PCN allergy, peritoneal dialysis, MF, alopecia areata
Onychauxis	Thickened, no dystrophy, yellowed	Elderly
No eponychium	No cuticle	Yellow-nail syndrome
Hypereponychium	Cuticular overgrowth = Samitz sign	Dermatomyositis
Eponychium hyperpigmentation	Hyperpigmented cuticle	Pellagra, porphyria cutanea tarda
Pits	Defect of dorsal proximal nail matrix	Psoriasis, alopecia areata, many more
Leukonychia	Defect of ventral proximal nail matrix	
Melanonychia	Distal lunular (ventral) matrix location	
Groove	Defect of proximal nail fold	Myxoid cyst
Verrucous nail bed		Incontinentia pigmenti
Racket nail	Transverse > longitudinal dimension	Scleroderma

[a] All nail defects except pits, which originate from the dorsal nail matrix, are from the ventral nail matrix.

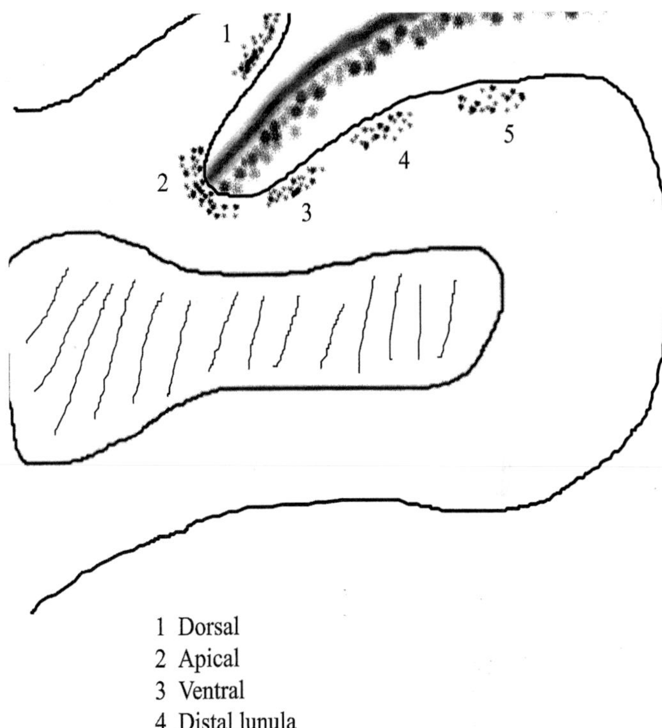

FIGURE 8–4
Drawing of nail matrix.

NICOTINIC STOMATITIS

- Fissuring plaque composed of umbilical nodules with central red spots, which are inflamed openings of salivary ducts.

DIFFERENTIAL DIAGNOSIS OF PEGGED TEETH

- Anhidrotic ectodermal dysplasia
- Incontinentia pigmenti
- Congenital syphilis

DIFFERENTIAL DIAGNOSIS OF PITTED TEETH

- Junctional EB (Herlitz)
- Tuberous sclerosis (48% of patients)
- Nevoid BCC syndrome (Gorlin syndrome)

TABLE 8–7
ECTOPIC SEBACEOUS GLANDS

Name	Location
Fordyce spots	Oral mucosa
Meibomian glands	Eyelids (open into follicle), primary source of sebaceous carcinoma
Zeiss glands	Eyelids (do not open into follicle)
Tyson glands	Penis
Montgomery tubercles	Nipples
Koplik spots	Altered sebaceous glands in measles
Moll glands	Eye: aprocine glands

SWEAT

Substances that have a higher concentration in sweat than in plasma.

- Lactate
- Ammonia
- Urea
- Amino acids (ornithine, serine, aspartate, citrulline)

TABLE 8–8
TYPES OF PAPILLAE (ON TONGUE)

Papillae	Location
Circumvallate	V-shaped groove (terminal sulcus)
Filiform	Numerous on dorsal tongue; dominant type
Fungiform	Tip + lateral margins; contain taste buds

TABLE 8–9
TYPES OF TONGUE

Type	Disease Association	Treatment
Smooth	Sprue	Underlying disorder
Black, hairy	Bacterial overgrowth	Brushing, trichloracetic acid, 40% urea rinses, 1% hydrogen peroxide
Geographic	Psoriasis	Reassurance
White or strawberry	Scarlet fever (initially red strawberry)	
Fissured/scrotal = lingua plicata	Melkersson-Rosenthal (which also includes facial paralysis and lip edema) Down syndrome	Surgery + intralesional triamcinolone acetonide (Kenalog)
Median rhomboid glossitis	Chronic candidiasis vs. developmental defect	Absence of filiform papillae

ACQUIRED TRICHOMEGALY (LENGTHENED EYELASHES)

- AIDS
- IFN-α_{2A} therapy (for non-Hodgkin lymphoma)
- Cyclosporine
- Chronic illness
- Kala-azar (Pitalnga sign)
- Malnutrition

DIFFERENTIAL DIAGNOSIS OF YELLOW-NAIL SYNDROME

Absence of eponychium (cuticle) is pathognomonic.

- Lymphedema (Milroy disease)
- Penicillamine
- Thyroid disease
- Bronchiectasis/lung disease
- Rheumatoid arthritis
- Malignancy

CHAPTER

9

DERMATOLOGIC SURGERY AND LASER THERAPY

TABLE 9–1
ANESTHETICS[a]

	Ester	Amide[b] (***i*** am an amide)
Anesthetic	Procaine (Novocaine) Chlorprocaine/cocaine Tetracaine (46 h) (longest-acting ester) Benzocaine D**i**bucaine (exception to the rule)	Bup**i**vacaine (Marcaine) (4–8 h, longest-acting) Et**i**docaine (4–6 h) Mep**i**vacaine (Carbocaine) (4–6 h) Pr**i**locaine (1–6 h) (methemoglobinemia in children) L*i*docaine (Xylocaine)
Metabolized by	Tissue (pseudocholinesterase)	Liver
Excreted by	Kidney	Kidney
Other	Cross-reacts with PABA	Allergy to amide is allergy to Paraben preservative Preservative-free amide (lidocaine) may be used

[a] "**i**" before -caine is evidence of an am**i**de.

[b] Amides rarely cause allergic reactions: "Amides are amigos (friends)."

TABLE 9–2
ANTIBIOTIC PROPHYLAXIS FOR SURGERY

	Skin Pathogen (1 h before, (6 h after)	Oral Pathogen (1 h before, 6 h after)
First-line	Cephalexin (1 + 0.5 g)	Amoxicillin (1.5 + 3 g)
Second-line	Dicloxacillin (1 + 0.5 g)	Erythromycin (0.5 + 1 g)
Third-line	Clindamycin (150 + 300 mg)	Clindamycin (150 + 300 mg)

CRYOSURGERY

- Liquid nitrogen = −195.8°C
- Carbon dioxide = −78.5°C
- Freon = +3.6 to −32°C
- Cryonecrosis = −25°C (benign lesions)
- Malignancy = −50°C (malignant lesions)

TABLE 9–3
DRESSINGS

Dressing	Characteristics
Alginates	Most absorptive
Hydrocolloids	Fibrinolytic, angiogenesis, inhibit keratinocyte migration, antibacterial
Hydrofilms	Occlusive, allow gas + water vapor
Hydrogel	Good for dry, painful wounds
Foams	Absorptive

EAR: SENSORY INNERVATION

- Superior helix: lesser occipital nerve
- Inferior helix + posterior ear: great auricular nerve
- External meatus/concha: vagus, auricular branch

TABLE 9–4
ELECTROSURGERY

Modality	Electrodes	Volts	Current	Waveform	Cutting vs. Coagulation[a, b]
AC Electrofulguration—pinpoint electrodessication; ball	1 (Hyfrecator)	↑	↓	Highly damped	Pure coagulation
AC Electrocoagulation; hemostat	2	↓	↑	Damped	Cutting and coagulation
AC Electrosection; sine wave	2	↓	↑	Slightly damped, continuous	Pure cutting
DC Electrolysis (makes sodium hydroxide at base of follicle)	2	↓	↓		

TABLE 9–4
ELECTROSURGERY (Continued)

Modality	Electrodes	Volts	Current	Waveform	Cutting vs. Coagulation
DC Electrocautery (heat stick)	ϕ	↓	↑		

[a] Pacemaker: electrodessication/fulguration with bursts of less than 5-s duration is acceptable; heat cautery is OK.
[b] Defribillator pacemaker: may trigger with any AC current device.

EPINEPHRINE

- Maximum time to blanching: 5–30 min
- Should not be used when biopsing mastocytosis lesion

ERB POINT

- 6 cm below ear/jawline junction
- Cranial nerve XI (spinal accessory), greater auricular nerve, and lesser occipital nerve susceptible to injury
- Transection of spinal accessory nerve affects trapezius muscle.

FACIAL ARTERIES

Internal Carotid	External Carotid
Supratrochlear	Infraorbital
Supraorbital	Facial
Infratrochlear	Maxillary
Dorsal nasal	Temporal
	Buccal
	Angular

FACIAL NERVE: BRANCHES IN ORDER

Mnemonic: Ted Zalinsky purchased/bought my car.

Temporal
Zygomatic
Posterior auricular (comes off first)
Buccal
Marginal mandibular
Cervical

- Dropped angle/corner of mouth caused by transected marginal mandibular (results in drooling).
- Inability to raise eyebrow caused by transected temporal branch.

FLAPS[a]

Rotation	Advancement	Transposition	Dog Ears	Pedicle
Simple	Simple	Rhombic	M-plasty (shorten scar)	Island
Bilateral	Bilateral	Limberg	Splasty	Paramedian
O to Z (double)	Burow triangle	Nasolabial		
Glabellar turndown	Helical	Labial-alar		
	A to T	Bilobed		
	V to T	Z-plasty (fix postsurgical lip lift)		
	U flap	(Paramedian)		
	O to U			
	Double (island)			

[a] Topical nitroglycerin can be used for flap tip that appears very white on follow-up.

GRAFT SURVIVAL

Dependent on the following:

1. Graft thickness: split-thickness skin grafts (STSGs) survive better than full-thickness skin grafts (FTSGs) because of little dermis.
2. Vascularity of recipient bed: if recipient is exposed cartilage or bone, graft does poorly.
3. Patient's nutritional status
4. Patient's smoking: this decreases viability
5. Contact between graft and vascular bed: treatment of hematoma/seroma is important.

INNERVATION

- Glabella and medial canthus—supratrochlear nerve
- Nasal tip—nasociliary nerve

JESSNER SOLUTION

- Resorcinol
- Salicylic acid
- Lactic acid
- Ethanol

TABLE 9–5
LASERS

Laser	λ (nm)[a]	Color	Chromophore	Mode
Excimer	193, 308, 351			Pulsed
Argon	488–514	Blue	Hb,[c] melanin	Continuous
Pigmented lesion dye	500–520	Green	Melanin	Pulsed
Copper	511, 578	Green	Hb, melanin	Semicontinuous
Krypton	521, 530, 568	Green	Hb	Continuous
Frequency-doubled Nd:YAG (KTP)	532		Melanin	Q-switch
Flash-lamp pulsed dye	585, 595, 600	Yellow	Hb	Pulsed
Gold vapor[b]	628	Red	Porphyrin	
Argon pumped dye[b]	630	Red	Porphyrin	Continuous
Q-switch ruby	694	Red	Melanin, tattoo	Q-switch
Q-switch alexandrite	755	Red	Melanin, tattoo	Q-switch
Titanium:sapphire	795		Melanin, tattoo	Picosecond
Diode	800			
Q-switch Nd:YAG	1,064	Infrared	Nonspecific	Q-switch
Holmium:YAG	2,100			
Erbium:YAG	2,940	Infrared	H_2O = 15- to 20-μm/pass	Continuous
CO_2	10,600	Infrared	H_2O = 25- to 50-μm/pass	Continuous

[a] Increased λ increases depth of penetration.
[b] Used for photodynamic therapy.
[c] Hb = hemoglobin.
Note: Laser resurfacing: reepithelization starts from appendages.

TABLE 9–6
LASER/EYE INTERACTIONS

λ (nm)	Structure Damaged	Laser	
<320	Cornea	Excimer	*All* lasers damage the retina except:
320–400	Lens	Excimer	• Nd:YAG, diode = lens + retina
400–700	Retina, choroids	Pulsed dye, Nd:YAG, ruby	• Excimer, Erbium:YAG, CO_2 = cornea
780–1400	Lens, vitreous, retina	Diode, Nd:YAG	
>1400	Cornea	Erbium:YAG, CO_2	

TABLE 9–7
LASER TREATMENT OF TATTOO PIGMENT

Tattoo Pigment	λ Absorbed (nm)	Lasers
Black, green	694–1064	Picosecond titanium:sapphire, 795 nm Q-switch ruby, 694 nm Q-switch alexandrite, 755 nm Q-switch Nd:YAG, 1064 nm
Red	510–532	Frequent-doubled Nd:YAG, 532 nm Flash lamp–pumped pulsed dye, 510 nm
Flesh-colored, white or iron-containing	Any	Ferric oxide converts to ferrous oxide, which turns color black

TABLE 9–8
LIDOCAINE

Mechanism	Decreased permeability to Na+
Standard concentration	1% = 10 mg/mL
Peak concentration	After tumescence = 4–8 h
Maximum dosage	4.5 mg/kg (no epinephrine) (~300 mg) 7 mg/kg (with epinephrine) (~500 mg) Tumescence: 35–65 mg/kg
Duration	30–60 min (no epinephrine) 2–3 h (with epinephrine)
Low toxicity	Perioral pallor, numbness, paresthesias
Medium toxicity	Nystagmus, slurred speech, hallucination
High toxicity	Cardiac arrest, coma
Death caused by	Respiratory arrest
Toxicity with	Tumescence + sertraline, flurazepam
Allergy	Occurs to parabens preservative, use preservative-free instead

PHENOL PEELS

Cardiac arrythmia is a potential side effect.

TABLE 9–9
PHOTODYNAMIC THERAPY (PDT)

Lasers	λ (nm)
Argon-pumped dye	450–630
Copper vapor	510–578
Gold vapor	628
Diode	770–850
Nd:YAG	690–1100

[a] Red light has greater penetration.

- works only on abnormal skin

TABLE 9–10
DRUGS USED IN PHOTODYNAMIC THERAPY

Drug	λ Absorbed (nm)
Porfimer sodium (Photofrin)	630–635
Aminolevulinic acid	630–635
Porphines, porphycenes	630
Phthalocyanines	650–700
Chlorines	>650
Benzoporphyrin derivate	690
N-Aspartyl-chlorine	664
Tin etiopurpurine	660
Lutetium texapyrine	732

AMINOLEVULINIC ACID (ALA)

- 20% (used for actinic keratoses) applied under occlusion bypasses rate-limiting step accumulating porphyrin IX.
- Porphyrin IX and light produces singlet oxygen: induces apoptosis, vascular damage, inflammatory response.
- DMSO, EDTA, and desferrioxamine enhance ALA penetration
- Heat and doxorubicin enhance photodynamic therapy.

SCALP LAYERS

- Epidermis
- Dermis
- Subcutis
- Galea aponeurotica
- Subgaleal space (best for undermining because it is relatively avascular)
- Pericranium

HEALING BY SECONDARY INTENTION

- Works best in concave aspects of ear, temple, eye, nose
- Works poorly (cosmetically) in convex areas such as the nose, lips, cheeks, chin, helix

TABLE 9–11
ABSORBABLE SUTURES

Suture	Brand	Configuration	Tensile Strength	Absorption	Reactivity
Gut	Plain	Twisted	1 week	90 days	High
Gut	Chromic	Twisted	3–4 weeks	90 days	High
Polyglactin	Vicryl	Braided	3–4 weeks	90 days	Low
Polyglycolic acid	Dexon	Braided	3–4 weeks	90 days	Low
Polydioxanone	PDS	Monofilament[a]	6–8 weeks	180 days	Low

[a] Monofilaments have high memory (low knot security) and are used in wounds because of the lower infection rate.

TABLE 9–12
NONABSORBABLE SUTURES

Suture	Configuration	Reactivity	Location
Silk	Braided/twisted	High	Mucosa
Mersilene (polyester)	Braided	Low	Mucosa
Polypropylene (prolene)	Monofilament	Low	Skin
Nylon	Monofilament	Low	Skin

TABLE 9–13
STITCHES

Stitch	Best for
Simple interrupted	Approximation of skin edge, minimal tension
Everted dermal	Approximation of deep dermis, reduction of dead space
Inverted dermal	Approximation of superficial dermis, hemostasis
Vertical mattress	Eversion of skin edges
Horizontal mattress	Tension of skin edges
Half-buried mattress	Tip stitch for flaps
Figure-of-eight	Hemostasis
Pulley stitch	Temporary reduction of tension
Purse string	Reduce defect size

TABLE 9–14
TATTOO PIGMENTS

Color	Pigment	Dermatitis
White	Titanium	
Yellow	Cadmium	Photosensitivity (yellow=color of sun!)
Green	Chromium or copper	
Blue	Cobalt	
Red	Mercury	Contact dermatitis
Purple	Manganese	
Black	Carbon	
Brown	Iron	

TABLE 9–15
TRIGEMINAL NERVE

Branch	Sensory Nerve
V_1 = ophthalmic	Supratrochlear
	Supraorbital
	Infratrochlear
	External nasal (tip)
V_2 = maxillary	Infraorbital
	Zygomatic
V_3 = mandibular	Buccal
	Auricolotemporal
	Mental

Notes: Anterior neck and mandibular area innervated by cervical plexus branches. Block mental nerve for lower lip excision.

TABLE 9–16
UV RADIATION[a,b]

Radiation	λ (nm)
UVC	<290
UVB	290–320
NBUVB	311
UVA-2	320–340
UVA-1	340–400
Visible	400–760
Soret	410

[a] Dead Sea has increased UVA.

[b] UV light has highest energy of sun's spectrum reaching earth (higher than visible or infrared).

TABLE 9–17
WOUND STRENGTH

Time after Wound	Percent Strength
2 weeks	5%
3 weeks	20%
1 month	50%
Final healing (unlimited time)	80%

CHAPTER 10

DERMATOPATHOLOGY

TABLE 10–1
DIFFERENTIAL DIAGNOSIS OF ACANTHOLYSIS

Lesion/Disease		Pathology/Clinical Manifestations	Gene Defect
Warty dyskeratoma	Pemphigus	"Tombstone" cells, intertriginous	
Acantholytic SCC	Grover	Older men, trunk	
Acantholytic AK	Darier	Corps ronds/ grains = dyskeratosis	*serca-2* gene (Ca^{2+}-dependent)
Focal acantholytic dyskeratoma	Hailey-Hailey	"Dilapidated brick wall"; intertriginous macerated fissuring	Mutations of ATPase pump gene affect desmosomal cadherins
		Darier: *ATP2A2* gene (chromosome 12)	Hailey-Hailey: *ATP2C1* gene

DIFFERENTIAL DIAGNOSIS OF ACQUIRED DIGITAL FIBROKERATOMA (PATHOLOGY)

- Supernumerary digit (nerve bundles at base of lesion)
- Amputation neuroma

HISTOLOGIC TYPES OF ACTINIC KERATOSIS

- Hypertrophic
- Bowenoid
- Atrophic
- Lichenoid
- Acantholytic
- Pigmented

Note: No parakeratosis over follicular orifice.

DIFFERENTIAL DIAGNOSIS OF AMORPHOUS EOSINOPHILIC MATERIAL

- Nodular amyloid
- Colloid milium
- Lipoid proteinosis
- Erythropoietic protoporphyria
- Gout

AMYLOID STAINS

- Congo red: polarized light → green birefringence (also seen in colloid milium).
- Fluorescent: thioflavin T (green/yellow), Phorwhite BBU.
- Crystal violet and methyl violet: metachromatic (red).
- PAS+/diastase-resistant (purple).
- Cotton dyes: Pagoda red, RIT scarlet No. 5, Sirius Red, Dylon.
- Differentiate primary and secondary amyloidosis: potassium permanganate ($KMnO_4$).
- Stain with $KMnO_4$, primary keeps birefringence, secondary loses it.

ASTEROID BODIES

Differential diagnosis of Splendori-Hoeppli phenomena: these are *not* pathognomonic.

- Central area made up of degenerated collagen.

Idiopathic	Mycobacteria	Fungi
NLD Necrobiotic xanthogranuloma Sarcoidosis Annular elastolytic granuloma	Tuberculosis Leprosy	Sporotrichosis *Histoplasma* *Cryptococcus* *Aspergillus* *Mucor/Zygomycetes*

Foreign Body		
• Beryllium (fluorescent bulbs)		
Parasites	**Graphite**	**Tumors**
• *Schistosoma*	Mercury Silicon/silica Polytef (Teflon) Zirconium (deodorants = axillae)	Cystic teratoma Fibrocystic mastopathy Fibroxanthosarcoma

DIFFERENTIAL DIAGNOSIS OF SUBCORNEAL BLISTERS

Common	Childhood	Other
Pemphigus foliaceous	Acropustulosis of infancy	Cutaneous *Candida*
Subcorneal pustular dermatosis	Erythema toxicum neonatorum (eosinophils)	Miliaria crystallina
Bullous impetigo/ Staphylococcal scalded skin syndrome	Transient neonatal pustular melanosis	Bullous tinea Pustular psoriasis IgA pemphigus

DIFFERENTIAL DIAGNOSIS OF BLISTERS (SUBEPIDERMAL CELL-POOR)

Common	Rare
PCT	Suction blister
EB	Bullous disease of renal failure
BP (cell-poor)	Bullous diabeticorum (lamina lucida split)
	Bullous amyloid
	Friction blister (usually intraepidermal)
	Coma bulla (eccrine gland necrosis)

DIFFERENTIAL DIAGNOSIS OF BLISTERS (SUBEPIDERMAL AND PMNs)

- DH
- Linear IgA/chronic bullous disease of childhood
- Bullous lupus
- BP/CP/HG
- EBA
- Bullous scabies
- Bullous mastocytosis (usually mast cells)

DIFFERENTIAL DIAGNOSIS OF CLEAR CELLS

- *Clear cell* acanthoma
- *Clear cell* hidradenoma (eccrine acrospiroma)
- *Clear cell* BCC or SCC
- *Clear cell* syringoma
- Trichilemmoma
- Balloon cell nevus
- Renal cell carcinoma

DIFFERENTIAL DIAGNOSIS OF COLLOID BODIES

- *Lichen* planus and variants (LPP)
- *Lichen* nitidus
- *Lichenoid* keratosis (LPLK)
- *Lichenoid* drug
- *Lichenoid* GVH
- Lupus
- Poikiloderma atrophicans vasculare
- GVH

DIFFERENTIAL DIAGNOSIS OF COMMA BODIES

- Benign cephalic histiocytosis
- +/– JXG

DIFFERENTIAL DIAGNOSIS OF POSITIVE CONGO RED STAINS

Green birefringence:

- Amyloid
- Colloid milium
- Lipoid proteinosis
- Porphyria

DIFFERENTIAL DIAGNOSIS OF CORNOID LAMELLA

- Porokeratosis
- Seborrheic keratosis
- Pachyonychia congenita
- Verruca vulgaris
- AK/Bowen's
- BCC

DIFFERENTIAL DIAGNOSIS OF CORPS RONDS

- Darier disease
- Grover disease
- Warty dyskeratoma
- Focal acantholytic dyskeratoma
- Lichen striatus

DIFFERENTIAL DIAGNOSIS OF CUTANEOUS HORN

- AK → SCC
- Seborrheic keratosis
- Filiform wart
- BCC
- Tricholemmoma
- Gout

TABLE 10–2
CYSTS (CILIATED VS. COLUMNAR)

Ciliated Cysts	Columnar	Ciliated	Clinical Site	Pathology
Cutaneous ciliated	+	+	Legs of black females	Like fallopian tubes (vulva)
Bronchogenic	+	+	Above sternal notch	Goblet cells, smooth muscle
Thyroglossal duct	+	+	Anterior neck, 1% malignant, moves with swallowing or tongue protrusion	Thyroid follicles, no smooth muscle
Branchial cleft		+	Preauricular to lateral neck	+/− Cartilage, lymphoid tissue around cyst wall
Median raphe	+		Glans penis	Pseudostratified columnar epithelium, like urethra

DIFFERENTIAL DIAGNOSIS OF DEEP TUMOR

Usually no epidermis on slide:

- Rheumatoid nodule
- Sclerosing lipogranuloma (paraffinoma)
- Giant cell tumor of tendon sheath
- Schwannoma
- Angiolipoma
- Myxoid liposarcoma
- Hibernoma
- Chondroid syringoma
- Angioleiomyoma
- Nodular fasciitis
- Leiomyoma

TABLE 10–3
DIFFERENTIAL DIAGNOSIS OF DERMAL PALLOR

Diagnosis	Contents in Dermis	Other Findings
Sweet Syndrome	Edema	Neutrophils, dust
PMLE	Edema	Lymphocytes, RBCs
Radiation	Altered collagen	Fibroblasts
Lichen sclerosus	Altered collagen	Fibroblasts, lymphocytes
Myxedema	Collagen splayed by mucin	Also cyst, mucocele, + focal cutaneous mucinosis
Pretibial	Goes from deep to superficial	
Papular	Spindled fibroblasts + mucin, looks like granuloma annulare	

DIFFERENTIAL DIAGNOSIS OF DESMOPLASTIC TRICHOEPITHELIOMA

- Desmoplastic trichoepithelioma
- Syringoma
- Metastatic adenocarcinoma
- Morpheaform BCC
- Microcystic adnexal carcinoma
- Scirrhous breast carcinoma ("indian file" pattern)

TABLE 10–4
APPEARANCE ON ELECTRON MICROSCOPY

Entity	Appearance
Molluscum	Virus = "dumbbell" shape
Eosinophils	Bilobed nucleus, granules = refractile crystals
Granular cell	"Bubbles in trash"
Langerhans cell	Birbeck "tennis racket" granules, convoluted nucleus
Merkel cell	***Vacuoles;*** extranuclear membrane-bound granules; occasional filaments, circular, desmosomes
Keratinocytes	"Stack of sticks" = filaments + desmosomes
Melanocytes	No filaments/desmosomes. Different colored granulars, slightly oval, pale cytoplasm
Mast cells	Same-sized, densely distributed "fingerprint" (lamellation) granules, *round* cell
Hair of anhidrotic ectodermal dysplasia	Longitudinal grooves
Uncombable hair syndrome	Longitudinal grooves
Amiodarone	Lamellated inclusions in endothelial cells

ENDOTHELIAL CELL MARKERS

- Factor VIII
- *Ulex europaeus*
- CD31 (most specific)
- CD34
- Vimentin
- Weibel-Palade body (electron microscopy)

DIFFERENTIAL DIAGNOSIS OF EOSINOPHILIC SPONGIOSIS

Mnemonic: HAPPIED

Herpes gestationis
Allergic contact/arthropod
Pemphigoid
Pemphigus
Incontinentia pigmenti
Erythema toxicum neonatorum
Drug

Subepidermal Blister	Intraepidermal Blister	Pediatric
BP/CP/HG	Pemphigus	Erythema toxicum neonatorum
DH	Subcorneal pustular dermatosis	Incontinentia pigmenti (has dyskeratotic cells)
Linear IgA	Grover (TAD)	
EBA		

Bugs	"Eosinophilic"	Infection	Other
Arthropod bite	Eosinophilic cellulitis (Wells)	Milker's nodule	Contact dermatitis drug reaction
Scabies	Eosinophilic pustular folliculitis		
Postscabetic nodule			
Larva migrans			

DIFFERENTIAL DIAGNOSIS OF EPIDERMOLYTIC HYPERKERATOSIS

Specific	Nonspecific
Epidermolytic hyperkeratosis	Normal skin
Linear epidermal nevus (ichthyosis hystrix)	Seborrheic keratosis
Vorner palmoplantar keratoderma	AK/Bowen
Epidermolytic acanthoma	SCC
	Flat wart

DIFFERENTIAL DIAGNOSIS OF ERYTHROPHAGOCYTOSIS

- Histiocytic cytophagic panniculitis (subcutaneous t-cell lymphoma = "beanbag" cells)
- Malignant histiocytosis

FACE BIOPSY WITH EOSINOPHILS

- Granuloma faciale
- Angiolymphoid hyperplasia with eosinophilia
- Follicular mucinosis

DIFFERENTIAL DIAGNOSIS OF FLAME FIGURES

- Wells syndrome
- Bullous pemphigoid
- Dermatophyte
- Arthropod bite
- Eczema / prurigo
- Dermal hypersensitivity reaction

DIFFERENTIAL DIAGNOSIS *OF* CASEATING GRANULOMAS

Caseating = cell-poor, central necrosis

Infectious	Idiopathic
• Mycobacteria (*M. tuberculosis*, *M. marinum*, *M. ulcerans*—Buruli ulcer) • Syphilis (gummatous)	Acne agminata

DIFFERENTIAL DIAGNOSIS OF EPITHELIOID/ NAKED GRANULOMAS

Infectious	"Granulomatous"	Other
Sarcoid Mycobacteria (*M. tuberculosis, M. marinum, M. leprae*—tuberculous leprosy)	Foreign-body granuloma Granulomatous rosacea Granulomatous cheilitis	• Metastatic Crohn **May Look Like Sarcoid** Beryllium (fluorescent bulbs) Zirconium (deodorant = axillae)
Leishmaniasis Deep fungal lesion Syphilis (late; secondary or tertiary)		Silica Aluminum Talc Paraffin

DIFFERENTIAL DIAGNOSIS OF PALISADING-NECROBIOTIC GRANULOMAS

- GA/NLD/rheumatoid nodule/annular elastolytic granuloma
- Foreign-body granuloma
- Necrobiotic xanthogranuloma
- Eruptive xanthoma (may appear like interstitial GA)
- May look like gout

DIFFERENTIAL DIAGNOSIS OF SUPPURATIVE GRANULOMAS

Bacterial	Fungal	Other
Actinomycosis	Blastomycosis	Foreign-body reaction to keratin
Botryomycosis	Chromomycosis	Follicular occlusion triad
Cat scratch disease/ tularemia	Coccidioidomycosis/ paracoccidioidomycosis	Halogenodermas
Mycobacteria	Sporotrichosis	
Lymphogranuloma venereum	Candidal infection	
Granuloma inguinale		

DIFFERENTIAL DIAGNOSIS OF GRANULOMAS AND VASCULITIS

Mnemonic: Walt

Wegener's/Winkelmann (associated with collagen vascular disease + rheumatoid arthritis)
Allergic granulomatosis (Churg-Strauss)
Lymphomatoid granulomatosis

Temporal arteritis

DIFFERENTIAL DIAGNOSIS OF GRENZ ZONE

- Acrodermatitis chronica atrophicans
- Granuloma faciale
- Lepromatous leprosy
- Leukemia cutis
- Lymphoma cutis (B-cell)
- Colloid milium

TABLE 10–5
DIFFERENTIAL DIAGNOSIS OF "GROUND GLASS" EOSINOPHILIC HISTIOCYTE

Clinical	Diagnosis
Arthritis mutilans	Multicentric reticulohistiocytosis
Solitary acral lesion	Reticulohistiocytic granuloma
Congenital	Congenital self-healing reticulohistiocytosis
Adenopathy	Sinus histiocytosis with massive lymphadenopathy = Rosai-Dorfman

TABLE 10–6
IMMUNOFLUORESCENCE

Linear	Granular	Perivascular
BP (roof) (C3)	LCV (IgG, IgM, C3)	Henoch-Schönlein purpura (IgA)
EBA (floor) (IgG)	Erythema elevatum diutinum	PCT (IgG)
CP (IgG, C3)	Henoch-Schönlein purpura (IgA)	
Linear IgA	Urticarial vasculitis	**Intercellular**
Herpes gestationis (C3)	DH (IgA at DEJ)	Pemphigus varieties
Paraneoplastic pemphigus (C3)	Degos (IgM, C3)	
Bullous LE (IgG)	DLE (IgG)	**Other**
PCT (IgG)	Pemphigus erythematosus (25%: IgG at DEJ)	Lichen planus: fibrinogen at DEJ/BMZ CREST = pepper-dot epidermis

DIFFERENTIAL DIAGNOSIS OF INTERFACE DERMATITIS

- EM/TEN: necrotic keratinocytes
- Acute GVHD: satellite necrosis
- Lupus/DM: perivascular infiltrates
- PLEVA/PLC: scale, parakeratosis, wedge infiltrate
- Lichen planus: wedge-shaped hypergranulosis
- Lymphocyte recovery: 7 days after BMT
- Fixed drug: eosinophils then melanophages
- Phototoxic dermatitis: basal layer necrosis
- Ashy dermatosis: melanophages
- Morbilliform drug
- Viral exanthem

DIFFERENTIAL DIAGNOSIS OF INTRAEPIDERMAL PUSTULES

Adults	Infants
Pustular psoriasis	Impetigo
Subcorneal pustular dermatosis	*Candida*
Pemphigus foliaceus/erythematosus	Scabies
Geographic tongue	Infantile acropustulosis
	Transient neonatal pustular melanosis
	Erythema toxicum neonatorum
	Incontinentia pigmenti

DIFFERENTIAL DIAGNOSIS OF SUPERFICIAL AND DEEP DERMAL INFILTRATES

Mnemonic: 5 L's

Lupus/Jessner
Lymphocytoma cutis
Lymphoma cutis/leukemia cutis
Light eruption (PMLE)
Lues (secondary syphilis)

DIFFERENTIAL DIAGNOSIS OF TUMID LUPUS

Tight superficial/deep perivascular/periappendegeal infiltrate; no epidermal Δ

- Jessner lymphocytic
- Erythema annulare centrifugum (deep)
- Pernio/chilblains (treat with calcium-channel blocker)
- Rarely lymphoma

LANGERHANS CELL MARKERS

- S-100
- CD1a
- ATPase
- Peanut lectin
- α-D-mannosidase

LICHENOID DERMATITIS

Interface change and band-like infiltrate

- Lichen planus and variants
- Lichen nitidus
- Lichenoid keratosis
- Lichenoid drug
- Lichenoid GVH
- Lupus
- CTCL
- Lues (secondary syphilis; psoriasiform lichenoid with plasma cells)

DIFFERENTIAL DIAGNOSIS OF LYMPHOID FOLLICLE

- Lymphocytoma cutis (pseudolymphoma)
- Arthropod bite
- Lupus panniculitis/profundus
- Lymphoma cutis
- Angiolymphoid hyperplasia with eosinophilia

TABLE 10–7
MAST CELL STAINS

Nonmetachromatic	Metachromatic (Secondary to Heparin)
Methylene blue	Toluidine blue (metachromatic)
Chloracetate esterase (Leder)	Giemsa (metachromatic)
	Azure A (metachromatic)

MARKERS OF MELANOMA

- S-100
- CCR7
- Vimentin
- CD68
- MART-1
- MIB-1
- HMB-45 (negative in desmoplastic MM)

MERKEL CELL: IMMUNOHISTOCHEMISTRY

- LMW cytokeratin 20 (paranuclear) negative in normal Merkel cells
- Neuron-specific enolase most specific; positive in normal merkels
- Chromogranin A
- Bombesin negative in Merkel cell, positive in small cell lung cancer
- Synaptophysin: cytoplasmic
- CD57
- CD44: extensive staining indicates poor prognosis
- Ber-EP4

DIFFERENTIAL DIAGNOSIS OF MUCINOSES

"Myxedema"	"Mucinosis"
Generalized myxedema (hypothyroidism)	Cutaneous focal mucinosis (LAMB)
Pretibial myxedema (hyperthyroidism, exophthalmos)	Follicular mucinosis
Scleromyxedema (treat with melphalan or IVIG)	Reticular erythematous mucinosis (REM)
Scleredema	

Other
• Myxoid cyst, mucopolysaccharidoses

MUCOPOLYSACCHARIDE STAINING

Acid	Neutral	Sulfated
H&E Giemsa Colloidal Fe Mucicarmine Alcian blue pH 2.5 Toluidine blue Methylene blue	PAS GMS	Aldehyde fuschin Alcian blue pH 0.5

DIFFERENTIAL DIAGNOSIS OF NEUTROPHILIC DERMATOSIS

Behçet
Bowel bypass syndrome
Cellulitis/erysipelas
EED
PG
Sweet syndrome
Rheumatoid arthritis
DH
Sneddon-Wilkinson disease
Pyostomatitis vegetans

PATHOLOGIC DIFFERENTIAL DIAGNOSIS OF NORMAL SKIN

- Amyloid (macular)
- Anetoderma
- Atrophoderma
- Café-au-lait spot
- Tinea versicolor
- Parapsoriasis
- Ichthyosis
- Cutis laxa
- Myxedema
- Accessory nipple
- Scleredema
- Dermatophyte
- CT nevus
- GVH
- Pretibial myxedema
- Scleroderma
- Scleromyxedema
- Urticaria
- Urticaria pigmentosa/mast cell disease

DIFFERENTIAL DIAGNOSIS OF PAGETOID SPREAD

- Paget disease
- Paget disease, extramammary
- Pagetoid reticulosis (Woringer-Kolopp)
- Podophyllin
- Melanoma
- Bowen disease
- Bowenoid papulosis
- Sebaceous carcinoma

TABLE 10–8
IMMUNOHISTOCHEMISTRY OF PAGET DISEASE

Pagetoid Differential Diagnosis	CEA	EMA	LMW Cytokeratin	HMW Cytokeratin	S-100	PAS	Mucin
Paget disease	−	+	+	−	+		
Extramammary Paget	+	+	−	−	−	+ diastase-resistant	+
Bowen	−	−	−	+	−		
Melanoma	−	−	−	−	+		
Eccrine tumors	+	+	−	−	−		
Adenocarcinoma	+	−	−	−	−		

DIFFERENTIAL DIAGNOSIS OF LOBULAR PANNICULITIS

- Weber-Christian
- Pancreatic
- Posttraumatic
- Physical
- Neonatal (sclerema neonatorum)
- Subcutaneous fat necrosis of newborn
- Granuloma annulare
- Infection/idiopathic
- Lupus profundus
- Lymphoma/leukemia
- Sarcoid
- α_1-Antitrypsin deficiency
- Lobular with vasculitis (erythema induratum)

DIFFERENTIAL DIAGNOSIS OF SEPTAL PANNICULITIS

- Scleroderma
- Erythema nodosum
- Eosinophilic fasciitis
- Necrobiosis lipoidica

TABLE 10–9
PANNICULITIS: SPECIFIC PATHOLOGIC FINDINGS

Panniculitis	Pathologic Finding
Erythema nodosum	Widened septa, giant cells
Cold	Needles
Poststeroid	Needles
Subcutaneous fat necrosis of the newborn	Needles
Subcutaneous T-cell lymphoma	Beanbag cells
Histiocytic cytophagic	Beanbag cells
Paraffinoma	Swiss cheese
Chemical	Swiss cheese
Lupus	Lymphoid follicles, lobular hyalinization, dermal mucin, waxy pink lipocytes, plasma cells
Pancreatic	Calcium (blue) surrounding pink feathery change, neutrophils
α_1-Antitrypsin deficiency	Ghost cells with calcium, "floating bubbles," neutrophils into dermis (lesions induced by trauma)
Lipodermatosclerosis	Stasis, cystic degenerations of fat, sclerotic changes, moth-eaten feathery membrane
Nodular vasculitis	Lobular, vasculitis, neutrophils, fat necrosis, liquefaction, very blue

PLASMA CELLS

- Kaposi sarcoma
- Lupus panniculitis
- Necrobiosis lipoidica diabeticorum
- Syringocystadenoma papilliferum
- Granulation tissue
- Acne keloidalis
- Oral biopsies
- Syphilis, mycloma

DIFFERENTIAL DIAGNOSIS OF PSAMMOMA BODY

- Meningioma
- Thyroid papillary carcinoma
- Nevocellular nevi
- Ovarian carcinoma
- Endosalpingiosis

DIFFERENTIAL DIAGNOSIS OF PSEUDOEPITHELIOMATOUS HYPERPLASIA

- Atypical mycobacterium
- Actinomycosis
- Blastomycosis (North American)
- Blastomycosis (South American = paracoccidiosis)
- Coccidioidomycosis
- Chromomycosis
- Protothecosis
- Sporotrichosis
- Halogenoderma
- Not cryptococcosis (usually in fat)

Noninfectious	Chronic Infection
• SCC	• Deep fungal
• KA	• Atypical mycobacteria
• Prurigo nodularis	• Leishmaniasis
• Halogenodermas	• Tertiary syphilis
• Chronic ulcer	• Granuloma inguinale
• Granular cell tumor	• Actinomycosis

DIFFERENTIAL DIAGNOSIS OF PSORIASIFORM DERMATOSES: PATHOLOGY

Characteristic	Diagnoses	Frequent	Occasional
Psoriasis	Lamellar ichthyosis	Contact dermatitis	Dermatophyte
PRP	Pellagra	Nummular dermatitis	*Candida*
Reiter	Acrodermatitis enteropathica	Seborrheic dermatitis	Scabies (crusted)
LSC	Necrolytic migratory erythema	Secondary syphilis	Bazex syndrome
ILVEN	Prurigo nodularis	MF	
		PR	

PUSTULOOVOID BODY

- Found in *granular cell tumor*
- Round eosinophilic inclusions made up of coalescing granules

REFRACTILE UNDER LIGHT MICROSCOPY

- Silica
- Starch
- Suture
- Silicone
- Lipid in xanthoma (doubly refractile)
- Wood
- Urate
- Amyloid stained with congo red
- Gelfoam

SIALOMUCIN

- Contains both acid and neutral mucopolysaccharides
- Stains with colloidal Fe and periodic acid–Schiff (PAS)

DIFFERENTIAL DIAGNOSIS OF SMALL ROUND CELL

- Small cell squamous cell
- Small cell melanoma
- Metastatic oat cell
- Carcinoid
- Merkel cell
- Extraskeletal Ewing sarcoma
- Retinoblastoma
- Neuroblastoma
- Rhabdomyosarcoma
- Leukemia/lymphoma

TABLE 10–10
DIFFERENTIAL DIAGNOSIS OF SPINDLE CELL

Spindle Cell Tumor	Immunohistochemistry
SCC	Cytokeratin
Spindle melanoma	S-100
AFX/MFH	Vimentin
DF	Factor 13a
DFSP	CD34
KS	Factor 8
Angiosarcoma	CD31
Leiomyosarcoma	Desmin

TABLE 10–11
DIFFERENTIAL DIAGNOSIS OF SPINDLE CELL: IMMUNOHISTOCHEMISTRY

	Vimentin	S-100	Cytokeratin
AFX	+	–	–
Melanoma	+	+	–
Spindle SCC	–	–	+

DIFFERENTIAL DIAGNOSIS OF SPLENDORE-HOEPPLI IMMUNE COMPLEX DEPOSITION

See also differential diagnosis of asteroid bodies, at the beginning of this chapter.

- Actinomycosis
- Mycetoma
- Sarcoid
- Botryomycosis
- Sporotrichosis

DIFFERENTIAL DIAGNOSIS OF SPONGIFORM PUSTULES

- Psoriasis
- Subcorneal pustular dermatosis
- Impetigo
- Geographic tongue
- *Candida*
- Reiter syndrome
- Halogenoderma

DIFFERENTIAL DIAGNOSIS OF CLUMPED TONOFILAMENTS

On electron microscopy:

- Epidermolytic hyperkeratosis
- Epidermolysis bullosa simplex, Dowling-Meara type
- Vorner palmoplantar keratoderma
- Erythrokeratoderma variabilis
- Friction blister

DIFFERENTIAL DIAGNOSIS OF TOUTON GIANT CELL

- Xanthomas
- Xanthoma disseminatum
- Juvenile xanthogranuloma
- Necrobiotic xanthogranuloma
- Histiocytosis X

ULEX EUROPAEUS

Immunohistochemical stain for

- Blood vessels (endothelial cells)
- Lymphatics

DIFFERENTIAL DIAGNOSIS OF GRANULOMATOUS VASCULITIS

- Syphilis
- Tuberculosis (papulonecrotic tuberculid)
- Leprosy
- Sarcoid

TABLE 10–12
SPECIAL STAINS

Stain	Application	Results
Actin	Muscle	
AFB/Fite/Ziehl-Neelsen	Acid-fast bacilli	Bacilli = red on all Fite good for leprosy Ziehl-Neelsen good for other mycobacteria
Alcian blue	Mucopolysaccharides	Blue
Alizarin red	Calcium	Red
Azure A	Mast cells	Metachromatically purple
Bodian	Nerve	
BRST-2	Metastatic breast cancer	
CEA	Extramammary Paget, eccrine tumors, adenocarcinoma	
Chloracetate esterase	Mast cells	Brilliant red granules
Colloidal iron	Mucopolysaccharides, glycoproteins	Blue
Congo red	Amyloid, colloid milium	Pink-smudgy, green birefringence
Crystal violet	Amyloid	Purplish-violet
Cytokeratin	Merkel, Paget, SCC, BCC	
Desmin	Muscle	
Dopa reaction	Cells with melanin	Gray-black
EMA	Paget (all), eccrine tumors, sebaceous glands	Red
Fontana-Masson	Melanin	Black
Foote	Reticulin fibers	Black
Fuelgen reaction	DNA	Magenta
Giemsa	Lymphoreticular elements, mast cells *Leishmania*	Metachromatically purple Blue

Gomori's aldehyde fuchsin	Elastic fibers	Black
Gram	Bacteria	Positive = blue, negative = red; positive has no lipid in wall
H&E	Routine	Nuclei blue, all else red
HMB-45	Melanocyte precursor, gp-100 protein	Positive in most MMs. Not always in desmoplastic MM
Leder (chloracetate esterase)	Mast cells	Brilliant red granules
Levaditi	Spirochetes	
Masson's trichrome	Fibrosis, leiomyoma	Collagen = green-blue
		Nuclei, muscle, + keratin = red
Mel-5	Antibody against tyrosinase (melanocytes)	Red (negative in amelanotic MM + albinism)
Methenamine silver	Fungi, parasites, Donovan bodies, Rhinoscl.	Black
Methyl-green-pyronin	RNA, DNA	RNA = pink, DNA = green
Mucicarmine	Adenocarcinomas	Mucin: red
	Cryptococcus	Capsule: red
	Rhinosporidium	
Oil Red O	Lipid	Red
Orcein-Giemsa	Elastic fibers (acid Orcein)	Black
	Amyloid	Blue
Periodic acid–Schiff (PAS)/ diastase	Fungi, parasites	Wall of organism: red
	Glycogen	Red on PAS, clear after diastase
	Basement membrane	Pink/red
	Cryoglobulinemia	Bright red
Peroxidase reaction	Myeloid leukemia	Uses benzidine to differentiate
Perls	Hemosiderin	Brown
Phorwhite BBU	Amyloid	Fluorescent

TABLE 10–12
SPECIAL STAINS (*Continued*)

Stain	Application	Results
Prussian blue/Perls	Hemosiderin/iron	Black
Phosphotungstic acid hematoxylin (PTAH)	Fibrin/muscle	Sarcoid (Asteroid bodies), infantile digital fibromatoses
S-100	Neuromelanocytic, Langerhans cells	
Scarlet red/Scharlack R	Lipid	Red
Schultz	Cholesterol esters	Tangier disease: green birefringence on polarized light
Snooks	Reticulin fibers	Black
Steiner	Spirochetes	
Sudan black B	Lipid	Black
Thioflavin T	Amyloid	Fluoresces blue-green
Thionine	Mucin	Metachromatically purple
Toluidine blue	Mast cells	Metachromatically purple
Verhoeff van Gieson	Arterial injury, elastic fiber	Blue-black (not in scar)
Vimentin	Melanocytes, sarcoma, lymphoma (fibroblast, endothelials, macrophages, smooth muscle)	
Von Kossa	Calcium	Black
Warthin-Starry	Spirochetes, Rochalimaea, rickettsiae, Donovan bodies (GI), *Bartonella*	Black

TABLE 10–13
BODIES

Name	Content	Disease Association
Asteroid	Pink STAR composed of collagen with radiations in granulomas. PTAH stain + (brown center + blue periphery)	Sarcoidosis Tuberculosis Sporotrichosis Granulomatous infiltrates Leprosy
Aschoff	Aggregates of histiocytes	Acute rheumatic fever
Banana	Schwann cells	Farber lipogranulomatosis (EM), ochronosis
Caterpillar	Pink necrotic material in blister roof in epidermis	Porphyria cutanea tarda
Cigar	Budding cells	*Sporothrix*
Civatte (hyaline/colloid/cytoid)	Necrotic keratinocyte	Lichen planus GVHD Amyloidoses Any interface dermatitis Lupus Poikiloderma
Comma		Benign cephalic histiocytosis Sinus histiocytosis LCH Congenital self-healing reticulohistiocytoma JXG

TABLE 10–13
BODIES (*Continued*)

Name	Content	Disease Association
Councilman	Cytoplasmic inclusions with cellular remnants	BCC Amyloid
Cowdry type A		HSV, VZV (EM)
Curvilinear	Lipid vacuoles	Farber lipogranulomatosis (EM)
Dorf balls	Pink amorphous globules in vessels	Kaposi sarcoma
Donovan		Granuloma inguinale
Farber		Farber lipogranulomatosis (EM)
Flame figures	Degranulated eosinophils within collagen	Wells BP Eczema Dermatophyte Arthropod Dermal hypersensitivity
"Floret" giant cells		Pleomorphic lipoma
Grenz zone		Granuloma faciale Lepromatous leprosy Leukemia cutis Lymphoma cutis (B-cell) Acrodermatitis chronica atrophicans Colloid milium

Guarnieri		Vaccinia Smallpox
Henderson-Patterson	Violet lobules in cytoplasm	Molluscum contagiosum virus
Kamino	Pale pink globules at the dermal papillae	Spindle + epitheliod nevus (60–80%) Melanoma (2%)
Lamellar		Fabry disease
Laminated dense		Congenital self-healing reticulohistiocytosis
Leishman	Tiny intracytoplasmic bodies/organisms	*Leishmania*
Lipschutz	Intranuclear eosinophilic inclusions	Herpes
Medlar (copper penny)		Chromoblastomycosis
Michaelis-Gutman	Intracellular calcified lamellated bodies	Malakoplakia
Mikulicz cells	Vacuolated cells (foamy cells with organisms)	Rhinoscleroma
Mulberry cells		Hibernoma
Myelin		Niemann-Pick disease (sphingomyelinase deficiency)
Negri		Rabies
Odland		Normal skin (EM)
Owl eye		CMV (EM)
Paschen	Variola virus	Smallpox

TABLE 10–13
BODIES (*Continued*)

Name	Content	Disease Association
Papillary mesenchymal	Blue islands with cap of differentiated stroma and condensation of blue cells appears like a "ball + claw"	Trichoepithelioma
Psammoma		Nevocellular nevus Cutaneous meningioma Thyroid papillary cancer Ovarian cancer Endosalpingiosis
Pustuloovoid body of Milian		Granular cell tumor
Residual	Pink globules in cytoplasm: collection of lysosomal granules	Granular cell tumor Sarcoid
Rocha-Lima	Endothelial pink-purple cytoplasmic inclusions	Verruga peruana
Russell	Plasma cell, no nucleus, with pink intracytoplasmic lobules	Rhinoscleroma Syphilis Plasma cell–rich infiltrate Multiple myeloma

Safety pin	Smear of *Calymmatobacterium granulomatis*	Granuloma inguinale
Schaumann	Concentric lamellated calcified bodies	Sarcoidosis Tuberculosis Granulomatous infiltrates Leprosy Berylliosis
School of fish	Seen in culture/smear of *Haemophilus ducreyi*	Chancroid
Tactoid	Whorled nerve-like body	Nevus
Tingible	Macrophages with blue-gray appearance	Pseudolymphoma (helps differentiate from lymphoma)
Verocay		Neurilemmoma Antoni A (schwannoma)
Virchow cells	Foamy histiocytes with globi of organisms	Leprosy
Warthin-Finley		Measles (rubeola)
Weibel-Palade		Endothelial cells (EM)
Zebra	Endothelial cells	Farber disease lipogranulomatosis (EM)

[a]EM = electron microscopy.

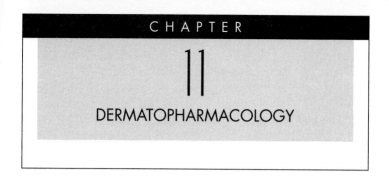

CHAPTER 11 DERMATOPHARMACOLOGY

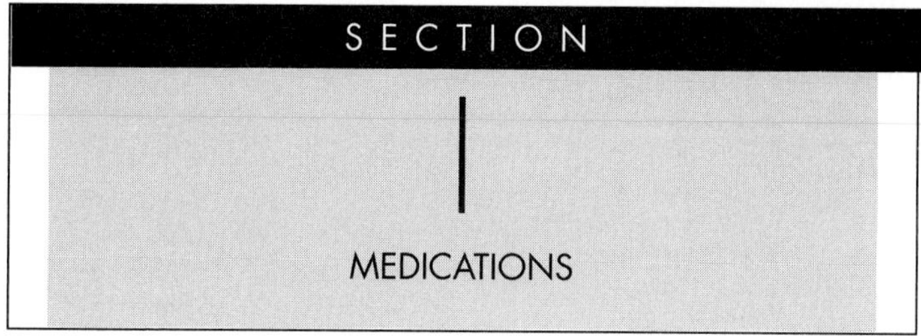

SECTION I MEDICATIONS

50S RIBOSOMAL UNITS ALL BOUND BY

- Clindamycin
- Chloramphenicol
- Macrolides

TABLE 11–1
ALDACTONE[a,b]

Cutaneous Side Effects		Systemic Side Effects
Subacute cutaneous lupus	Hypertrichosis	Hyperkalemia
Lichenoid	Raynaud	Gynecomastia
Erythema annulare centrifugum		

[a] Mechanism: Inhibits testosterone receptor and inhibits androgen synthesis.
[b] Contraindication: Cyclosporine.

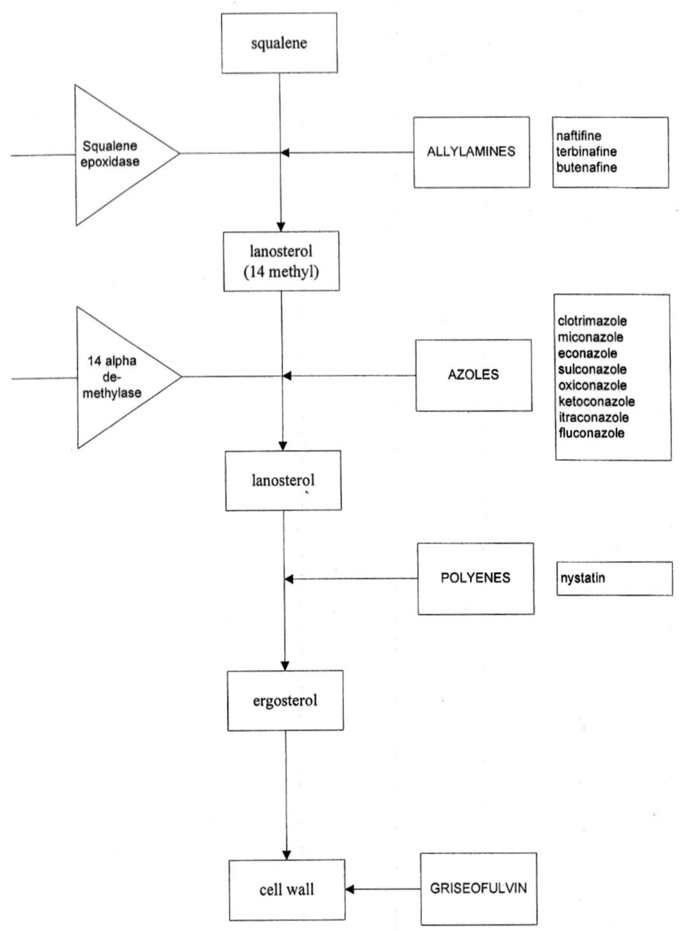

FIGURE 11–1
Antifungal pathway.

SIDE EFFECTS OF AMINOGLUTETHIMIDE

- Capillaritis (purpura simplex)
- Pustular psoriasis
- Lupus

SIDE EFFECTS OF AMIODARONE

- Slate-gray facial hyperpigmentation, photodistributed
- Linear IgA

TABLE 11–2
ANTIFUNGALS

Medication	Target	Mechanism	Factoide
Griseofulvin	Dermatophytes (not yeast)	Inhibits microtubule formation	Needs fatty meal/milk
Ketoconazole	Dermatophytes, yeast	Inhibits 14α demethylase	Fungistatic
Itraconazole	Dermatophytes, yeast, molds	Inhibits 14α demethylase	Needs acidic milieu
Fluconazole	Yeasts, dermatophytes	Inhibits 14α demethylase	
Lamisil	Dermatophytes, +/− yeasts	Inhibits squalene epoxidase	Fungicidal
Ciclopiroxo-lamine	Dermatophytes, yeast	Inhibits iron-dependent enzymes, ↓respiratory function, ↓nutrient uptake, ↑cell permeability	
Amphotericin B	All fungi	Inhibits ergosterol	Fungicidal

TABLE 11–3
ANTIHELMINTHICS

Drug	Action
Albendazole	Inhibits microtubules; worms migrate through mouth and nose
Diethylcarbazine (DEC)	Mazotti reaction in patients with onchocerciasis → fever, headache, eyes, pruritus
Ivermectin	Selectively binds worms' chloride ion channels, leading to paralysis
Mebendazole	Inhibits worms' microtubule formation and glucose uptake
Praziquantel	Alters worms' (usually schistosome) cell permeability (Biltricide)
Thiobendazole	Inhibits fumarate reductase

SIDE EFFECTS OF ANTIHISTAMINES

Doxepin blocks both H_1 (highest affinity) and H_2 antihistamine receptors.

SIDE EFFECTS OF ANTIPSYCHOTICS

- Photo-induced hyperpigmentation
- Tardive dyskinesia

SIDE EFFECTS OF ANTIRETROVIRALS

- Potent cytochrome P450 3A4 *inhibitors;* also increase rifampin levels
- Associated with partial lipodystrophy
- Indinavir: increased herpes zoster

SIDE EFFECTS OF AZT (ZIDOVUDINE)

- Blue lunula
- Hyperpigmented nails
- Anemia/bone marrow suppression

TABLE 11–4
ANTIVIRALS

Drug	Side Effects
Cidofovir[a]	Nephrotoxic
Famciclovir	Metabolite = penciclovir
Foscarnet	Mucosal ulcerations Electrolyte imbalance leads to seizures Renal toxicity
Ganciclovir	Neutropenia Irreversible pancytopenia Neurotoxicity (higher with Imipenem)
Ribavirin	Teratogenic for 6 months after use Hemolytic anemia Rash
Sorivudine	Contraindicated with 5-fluorouracil (5-FU)
Valacyclovir	Thrombocytopenic purpura Hemolytic-uremia syndrome Contraindicated in immunosuppressed patients

[a] Cidofovir 3% cream successfully treats plantar warts.

TABLE 11–5
ASCOMYCIN[a]

Uses		Side Effects
Atopic Dermatitis	Psoriasis	Stinging/burning

[a] Mechanism: Ascomycin is macrolactam that binds to cytosolic macrophilin-12 (FKBP-12), which inhibits IL-2 receptor.

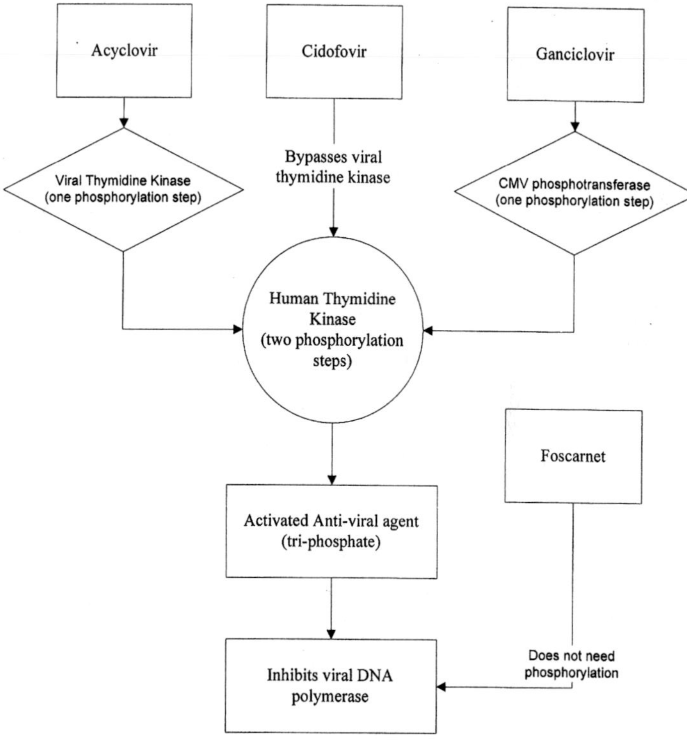

FIGURE 11–2
Antiviral pathway.

AZATHIOPRINE

Azathioprine takes effect in 4–6 weeks when used to treat an immunobullous reaction.
Mechanism: Azathioprine is a purine analog inhibiting DNA/RNA synthesis.
Contraindications: Allopurinol inhibits xanthine oxidase metabolic pathway (reduce azathioprine dose to one-third).
Reasons: Thiopurine methyltransferase deficiency inhibits TPMT metabolic pathway.

- Lesch-Nyhan syndrome inhibits HGPRT metabolic pathway.
- Azathioprine is a prior alkylating agent.
- Captopril increases the risk of leukopenia.

TABLE 11–6
AZATHIOPRINE

Cutaneous Side Effects	Systemic Side Effects	
Raynaud phenomenon Pellagra-like symptoms	Hepatitis Pancreatitis	Bone marrow suppression Lymphoma Opportunistic infections

SIDE EFFECT OF β-LACTAMS

Inhibit cell wall synthesis

SIDE EFFECTS OF TRIMETHOPRIM-SULFAMETHOXAZOLE (BACTRIM)

- Nephrolithiasis
- Sweet syndrome
- Fixed drug reaction
- Cholestatic hepatitis

TABLE 11–7
BASILIXIMAB[a]

Uses		Systemic Side Effects
Treatment of psoriasis	Prophylaxis of organ rejection	Gastrointestinal

[a] Mechanism: Basiliximab is a chimeric human/mouse monoclonal antibody for the IL-2 receptor (α-chain).

TABLE 11–8
BLEOMYCIN[a]

Cutaneous Side Effects		Systemic Side Effects
Raynaud phenomenon/ scleroderma Neutrophilic eccrine hidradenitis	Flushing Reversible penile calcifications	Pulmonary fibrosis (↑ with GCSF)
Hyperpigmentation: flagellate, striae, nail (banding), palmar crease	Acral erythema Toxic epidermal necrolysis	Anaphylaxis Pneumonitis

[a] Mechanism: Bleomycin binds DNA, inhibiting DNA synthesis (there is also some inhibition of RNA and protein synthesis).

TABLE 11–9
BUSULFAN[a]

Cutaneous Side Effects		Systemic Side Effects
"Dusky" bronze hyperpigmentation Brownish lunula and nail plate (longitudinal bands) Porphyria cutanea tarda	Gingival linear pigmentation Vasculitis Erythema nodosum	Bone marrow toxicity Pulmonary toxicity (fibrosis)

[a] Mechanism: Busulfan is a bifunctional alkylating agent.

CANTHARIDIN

Mechanism: Cantharidin is a phosphodiesterase inhibitor.

TABLE 11-10
CARMUSTINE (BCNU) AND FOTEMUSTINE/LOMUSTINE[a]

Cutaneous Side Effects		Systemic Side Effects
Flushing (including conjunctiva) Hyperpigmentation under ECG pads Telangiectasia	Lomustine: neutrophilic eccrine hidradenitis Fotemustine: serpentine supravenous hyperpigmentation Conjunctival suffusion	Bone marrow toxicity Pulmonary toxicity (fibrosis)

[a] Mechanism: Carmustine (BCNU) and fotemustine/lomustine alkylate both RNA and DNA.

SIDE EFFECT OF CEFACLOR

Serum sickness (onset 2–3 weeks after first dose)

TABLE 11–11
CLASSIFICATION OF CHEMOTHERAPEUTIC MEDICATIONS

ALKYLATING AGENTS	ANTIMETABOLITES
(not cell cycle–specific, bone marrow suppression)	*Purine Analogs*
• Busulfan	6-Mercaptopurine (6-MP)
• Carmustine (BCNU) + Fotemustine/lomustine/semustine (nitrosureas)	6-Thioguanine
Chlorambucil (nitrogen mustard)	Azathioprine
Cisplatin (and carboplatin)	Cladribine (leustatin)
Cyclophosphamide + ifosfamide (nitrogen mustard)	Fludarabine
Dacarbazine	Methotrexate (by inhibiting DHFR)
Mechlorethamine (nitrogen mustard)	*Pyrimdine Analogs*
Melphalan (nitrogen mustard)	Methotrexate (is also a thymidine analog)
Thiotepa (nitrogen mustard)	5-Fluorouracil (5-FU) + Floxuridine (FUDR)
	ARA-C (cytarabine)
	Other
	• Tegafur
ANTIBIOTICS	**MISCELLANEOUS**
Bleomycin	Docetaxel
Dactinomycin	Etoposide (VP-16)
Daunorubicin (and idarubicin)	Hydroxyurea
Doxorubicin	L-asparaginase
Mithramycin/plicamycin	Mitotane
Mitomycin C	Paclitaxel
Mitoxantrone	Procarbazine
Pentostatin	Vinca alkaloids

TABLE 11–12
CHEMOTHERAPEUTIC DRUG MECHANISMS (PRIMARILY INHIBITING SYNTHESIS OF DNA VS. RNA)

Primarily Inhibit DNA Synthesis		Inhibit RNA Synthesis (to a degree)
6-Mercaptopurine	6-Thioguanine	Azathioprine (both)
Azathioprine (both)	Cladribine	5-FU (partial)
Fludarabine	Methotrexate	Bleomycin (partial)
5-FU	Cytarabine	Dactinomycin (primarily)
Bleomycin	Daunorubicin	Doxorubicin (both)
Doxorubicin (both)	Mitomycin	Mithramycin/Plicamycin
Pentostatin	Hydroxyurea	Pentostatin (partial)
		Procarbazine[a]

[a] Procarbazine also inhibits protein synthesis.

TABLE 11–13
CHLORAMBUCIL[a]

Cutaneous Side Effects		Systemic Side Effects
Neutrophilic eccrine hidradenitis Hypersensitivity reactions	Acute intermittent porphyria Toxic epidermal necrolysis	Tonic-clonic seizures in children Leukemia/bone marrow toxicity

[a] Mechanism: Chlorambucil is a bifunctional alkylating agent (nitrogen mustard type).

TABLE 11–14
CISPLATIN[a]

Cutaneous Side Effects		Systemic Side Effects
70%: patchy hyperpigmentation, including extremities, nails, sites of pressure, hair color change, mucosa Leukonychia Inflammation of actinic keratoses	Acral erythema + flushing Porphyria Exfoliative dermatitis	Ototoxicity Bone marrow toxicity Renal toxicity

[a] Mechanism: Interstrand DNA cross links, not cell cycle-specific.

TABLE 11–15
CLADRIBINE (LEUSTATIN)[a]

Cutaneous Side Effects	Systemic Side Effects
Toxic epidermal necrolysis	Bone marrow, neurotoxicity, and nephrotoxicity

[a] Mechanism: Purine analog; disrupts cellular metabolism and impairs DNA synthesis and repair.

TABLE 11–16
CLOFAZIMINE

Cutaneous Side Effects		Systemic Side Effects	
Red-brown pigment in lesions + secretions Edema	Nail changes Xerosis Exacerbation of vitiligo	Bowel crystal deposition Fatal enteropathy Splenic infarction	Eosinophilic enteritis Cramping

CORTICOSTEROIDS

- Methylprednisolone has least salt/water-retaining effect (least mineralocorticoid effect)
- Prednisone is safest steroid in pregnancy
- Avoid systemic steroids in amyopathic dermatomyositis
- Alternate-dose steroid does not reduce likelihood of osteoporosis or cataracts
- Steroid receptor is in nucleus of cell

CYCLOPHOSPHAMIDE (CYTOXAN) AND IFOSFAMIDE

Mechanism: Alkylate purine DNA base pairs, thereby inhibiting B and T cells (nitrogen mustard type).

Interactions and why:

- Allopurinol, cimetidine, and chloramphenicol increase cyclophosphamide levels by inhibiting metabolism.
- Increase the toxicity of doxorubicin.
- Decrease the levels of digoxin because digoxin absorption is reduced.
- Not given with mechlorethamine.

TABLE 11–17
CYCLOPHOSPHAMIDE (CYTOXAN) AND IFOSFAMIDE

Cutaneous Side Effects		Systemic Side Effects
Hyperpigmentation: generalized or patchy of palms, soles, teeth + gingival (permanent)	Flare of dermatitis herpetiformis with doxorubicin + vincristine	Azoospermia/amenorrhea
Porphyria cutanea tarda + acute intermittent porphyria	Acral erythema + flushing	Acute myelogenous leukemia
Nails: transverse/horizontal bands/ridging	Hair color change: light red to black	Non-Hodgkin lymphoma
Vasculitis	UV recall	Hemorrhagic cystitis (caused by acrolein metabolite)
Neutrophilic eccrine hidradenitis	Ifosfamide: nail + skin hyperpigmentation, particularly under occlusion (ECG pads)	Bladder cancer
		Anaphylaxis/angioedema

CYCLOSPORINE (CyA)

Binds to cylophilin + calmodulin, stopping NFAT dephosphorylation; blocks IL-2 trancription.

Mechanism: Metabolized by cytochrome P450 (levels decreased by CYP inducers).

Contraindications:

- ACE inhibitors, potassium-sparing diuretics; trimethoprim-sulfamethoxazole (Bactrim) increases renal toxicity.
- CyA causes decreased clearance leading to increased levels of digoxin, statins, and prednisone via cytochrome P450.
- Retinoids: raise CyA levels.
- Terbinafine: lower CyA levels.

TABLE 11–18
CYCLOSPORINE

Cutaneous Side Effects	Systemic Side Effects	
Gingival hyperplasia Trichomegaly Hirsutism	↑K, ↓Mg, ↑uric acid, ↑triglycerides Hypertension (treat with calcium-channel blockers) Tremors Arthralgia	Paresthesias Proteinuria Myalgia Nephrotoxic

TABLE 11–19
CYTARABINE (ARA-C)[a]

Cutaneous Side Effects		Systemic Side Effects
Transverse leukonychia Inflammation of seborrheic and actinic keratoses Toxic epidermal necrolysis	Acral erythema Vasculitis Neutrophilic eccrine hidradenitis	Chemical arachnoiditis CNS toxicity (with coadministration of dexamethasone) Sweet syndrome

[a] Mechanism: S-phase–specific: Pyrimidine analog causes chain termination, inhibiting DNA polymerase.

TABLE 11–20
MNEMONIC FOR CYTOCHROME P450 INDUCERS

Mnemonic	The BAGIR—induces you to give money
B	Barbiturates
A	Anticonvulsants
G	Griseofulvin
I	Isoniazid
R	Rifampin

CYTOCHROME P450 3A4 INDUCERS[a]

Anticonvulsants	Antibacterial	Other	Foods
Barbiturates	Isoniazid	Nefazadone	Brussels sprouts
Carbamazepine	Nafcillin	Dexamethasone	Cabbage
Dilantin	Rifampin[b]	Griseofulvin	Charbroiled foods
Ethosuximide		Octreotide	Tobacco/chronic alcoholism

[a] Induction occurs after delay of days to weeks because it requires increased protein synthesis.
[b] Rifampin is the most potent inducer.

CYTOCHROME P450 3A4 INHIBITORS[a,b]

Inhibition occurs immediately, since it is based on competitive enzyme inhibition and does not require new enzyme synthesis.

Antibiotics	Antifungals	Cardiac	Other	Other
Bactrim	Azoles (not fluconazole)	Propranolol	Allopurinol	Fluoxetine/ SSRIs
Erythromycin, clarithromycin		Diltiazem	Cimetidine	Quinine
Fluoroquinolones		Verapamil	Oral contraceptives	Protease inhibitors
Flagyl		Nifedipine	Grapefruit juice	Tacrolimus
			Furosemide	INH (is both)
			Omeprazole	Ticlopidine
			Amiodarone	Interferon gamma

[a] Ketaconazole is the most potent inhibitor.
[b] Azoles/erythromycin + terfenadine/astemizole = prolonged QT duration then torsades de pointes.

CYTOCHROME P450 3A4 (TARGET DRUGS)

Drug levels that are frequently altered by concurrent medication. This is not a complete list.

Digitalis	Phenytoin	Dapsone
Warfarin	Oral contraceptives	Tricyclics
Lithium	Quinidine	Theophylline
Cyclosporine	Prednisone	Methotrexate

TABLE 11–21
DACARBAZINE[a]

Cutaneous Side Effects		Systemic Side Effects
Nail hyperpigmentation Fixed drug eruption	Inflammation of actinic keratoses Phototoxicity + flushing	Bone marrow toxicity Hepatic necrosis

[a] Mechanism: Either (1) inhibits DNA synthesis as a purine analog or (2) alkylates; used for metastatic melanoma.

TABLE 11–22
DACTINOMYCIN (ACTINOMYCIN D)[a]

Cutaneous Side Effects		Systemic Side Effects
Sterile folliculitis (mimics diffuse emboli) Acne Diffuse melanosis Supravenous serpentine hyperpigmentation	Bullous pemphigoid (with methotrexate) Phototoxicity Inflammation of actinic keratoses	GI and bone marrow toxicity

[a] Mechanism: Intercalates between G bases of DNA inhibiting RNA synthesis.

TABLE 11–23
DAPSONE: SIDE EFFECTS[a]

Dose-Related	Adverse Erythema Annulare Centrifugum (Idiosyncratic)	
Methemoglobinemia[b,c] Hemolysis of old RBCs due to ↓ glutathione (check hematocrit and reticulocyte count)	Agranulocytosis Psychosis Neuropathy (motor) Hypoalbuminemia	With leprosy → fatal mono-like disease Photodistributed bullous Erythema annulare centrifugum Cholestatic jaundice/ hepatitis optic atrophy

[a] Interactions: Bactrim, probenicid, and methotrexate raise dapsone levels; rifampin decreases dapsone levels.

[b] Reduce methemoglobinemia by coadministering cimetidine.

[c] Treat methemoglobinemia with methylene blue.

TABLE 11–24
DAUNORUBICIN AND IDARUBICIN[a]

Cutaneous Side Effects		Systemic Side Effects
Sun-exposed, hyperpigmentation	Leukonychia	Myocardial toxicity
Polycyclic scalp pigmentation	Acral erythema	Congestive heart failure
Brown-black horizontal nail bands	Folliculitis (liposomal form)	Myelosuppression

[a]Mechanism: Intercalate DNA base pairs and inhibit topoisomerase II, leading to breaks in ssDNA and dsDNA.

SIDE EFFECTS OF DIETHYLSTILBESTROL (DES)

- Acanthosis nigricans
- Hirsutism
- Lupus
- Porphyia cutanea tarda

DIHYDROXYACETONE

Ingredient in self-tanning preparations.

TABLE 11–25
DOCETAXEL (TAXOTERE)[a]

Cutaneous Side Effects		Systemic Side Effects
Pigmentation under ECG pads	Nail pigmentation	Severe hypersensitivity reactions
Acral erythema + flushing	Inflammation of actinic keratoses	
Scleroderma-like reaction		Hepatotoxicity
		Severe fluid retention

[a]Mechanism: Inhibits proper microtubule function.

TABLE 11–26
DOXORUBICIN (ADRIAMYCIN)[a]

Cutaneous Side Effects		Systemic Side Effects
Hyperpigmentation: (1) palmar hands, creases + dorsal hands (2) blue-gray on face, neck, shoulders Longitudinal + vertical blue nail bands Mucosal black pigmentation Dermatitis herpetiformis with cytoxan + vincristine Sticky skin with ketoconazole Black hair changes to red when given with bleomycin and vincristine	Acral erythema Phototoxic inflammation of actinic keratoses Toxic epidermal necrolysis Allergic contact (topical) dermatitis Neutrophilic eccrine hidradenitis Flushing	Colon ulceration + necrosis Myelosuppression Irreversible cardiomyopathy Congestive heart failure

[a] Mechanism: Intercalates DNA double helix, inhibiting DNA synthesis, RNA synthesis, and DNA repair.

TABLE 11–27
ETANERCEPT[a]

Uses		Side Effects
Psoriatic arthritis Rheumatoid arthritis	Severe psoriasis	Lupus flare 37% injection site reactions

[a] Mechanism: Fusion protein: recombinant TNF receptor and Fc fragment of IgG1 = competitive inhibitor of TNF-α.

SIDE EFFECTS OF ETHAMBUTOL

- Red-green color blindness
- Scotoma

TABLE 11–28
ETOPOSIDE (VP-16)[a]

Cutaneous Side Effects		Systemic Side Effects
Pigmentation of nail beds + fingers Acral erythema + flushing	UV recall pathology: "starburst keratinocyte" = podophyllin	Myelosuppression

[a] Mechanism: Podophyllin-derived: interacts with DNA topoisomerase II, causing DNA breaks = metaphase arrest.

TABLE 11–29
FLUDARABINE (ARA-A)[a]

Cutaneous Side Effects	Systemic Side Effects	
Inflammation of SCCs	CNS toxicity: blindness, coma, death Fatal pulmonary toxicity with pentostatin	Autoimmune hemolytic anemia

[a] Mechanism: Purine analog (i.e., vidarabine) inhibits DNA synthesis (DNA polymerase and primase, RNA reductase).

TABLE 11–30
FLUOROURACIL (5-FU) AND FLOXURIDINE (FUDR)[a,b]

Cutaneous Side Effects		Systemic Side Effects
Sun-exposed + localized hyperpigmentation	Acral erythema	Teratogenicity
Supravenous serpentine hyperpigmentation	Phototoxic flushing	
Flagellate + reticulate hyperpigmentation		
Hyperpigmentation of nails (blue), mucosa (tongue/conjunctiva)	Inflammation of actinic keratoses	
UV recall		
Toxic epidermal necrolysis	Folliculitis	

[a] Mechanism: Pyrimidine analog; inhibits thymidine synthesis, which inhibits DNA synthesis (incorporation into which then causes some inhibition of RNA synthesis).
[b] Contraindications: Sorivudine increases bone marrow toxicity.

SIDE EFFECTS OF FLUOXYMESTERONE

- Furunculosis
- Hirsutism
- Acne

TABLE 11–31
FLUTAMIDE[a]

Cutaneous Side Effects		Systemic Side Effects
Photoallergy	Flushing	Bone marrow toxicity Pulmonary toxicity (fibrosis)

[a] Mechanism: Antiandrogen; acts by inhibiting uptake and effect of androgens in target tissues.

TABLE 11–32
FOSCARNET[a]

Cutaneous Side Effects		Systemic Side Effects
16% oral ulcerations	5–28% of uncircumcised men have penile ulcerations	Electrolyte imbalances lead to seizures Renal toxicity

[a] Mechanism: Inhibits viral DNA/RNA polymerase and reverse transcriptase.

SIDE EFFECTS OF FUROSEMIDE

- Pseudoporphyria
- Phototoxicity
- Lichenoid reactions
- Bullous pemphigoid

GOECKERMAN THERAPIES

- Standard: 2–5% tar bath qd, excess tar removed, then UVB
- Modified (Ingram): tar bath qd (120 mL of liquor carbonis detergent with 80 mL of water), then UVB, followed by anthralin paste, talcum powder

TABLE 11–33
SIDE EFFECTS OF GOLD

Cutaneous	Systemic	
Lichen planus Pityriasis rosea Stomatitis Erythema annulare Centrifugum	Hepatic Keratitis + corneal ulcerations Thrombocytopenia + Leukopenia Subacute cutaneous lupus	Aplastic anemia Eosinophilia Pulmonary fibrosis

SIDE EFFECTS OF HYDROQUINONE

Pigmented colloid milium and ochronosis

SIDE EFFECTS OF HYDROXYCHLOROQUINE

- Retinopathy (scotoma)
- Corneal opacities
- Neuromuscular eye changes

TABLE 11–34
HYDROXYUREA[a]

Cutaneous Side Effects		Systemic Side Effects
Hyperpigmentation, more at pressure areas	Acral erythema	Leukemia
Diffuse dark nail & mucosal pigmentation	Dermatomyositis (long-term therapy)	Megaloblastic anemia
Black tongue	Fixed drug reaction	
Atrophic LP-like + lichenoid eruptions	Lupus	
Phototoxicity reaction	Telangiectasia	
Vasculitis	Poikiloderma, dorsal hands	
Ankle ulcers		
Palmoplantar keratoderma + nail changes		

[a] Mechanism: Inhibits RNA reductase preventing DNA synthesis and repair; S phase–specific.

SIDE EFFECTS OF INTERLEUKIN-2 (IL-2)

- Capillary leak syndrome
- Stomatitis
- Erythema nodosum
- Telogen effluvium
- Ulceration
- Exacerbation of psoriasis
- Linear IgA disease
- Scleroderma

SIDE EFFECTS OF INTERLEUKIN-1 (IL-1)

- Depression
- Fever
- Nausea and vomiting

TABLE 11–35
IMIQUIMOD[a,b]

Uses		Side Effects
HPV infections	Superficial BCCs	Irritation often leads to infection
Actinic keratoses	HSV infections	Contraindicated in renal transplant patients

[a] Resiquimod, next generation, more potent.

[b] Mechanism: Enhances production of IFN-α, TNF-α, and IL-12.

TABLE 11–36
INFLIXIMAB (REMICADE)[a]

Uses		Systemic Side Effects
Crohn disease Rheumatoid arthritis	Pyoderma gangrenosum Psoriasis	Infusion-related: fever/chills/rigors/urticaria/edema Hyper/hypotension

[a] Mechanism: Chimeric monoclonal antibody for TNF-α.

TABLE 11–37
SIDE EFFECTS OF INTERFERONS[a]

Interferons	Interferon α	Interferon β	Interferon γ
Exacerbate psoriasis + oral HSV Radiation enhancement CNS abnormalities/depression/psychosis Cardiomyopathy Flu-like symptoms Inflamed nasal mucosa	Spastic diplegia (2A) Trichomegaly (2A) Alopecia exacerbate dermatitis herpetiformis Linear IgA disease Lichenoid eruption with ribavirin	Thrombosis at injection site Rhabdomyolysis	Linear IgA disease

[b] α2B or alfacon-1 used for hepatitis C.

SIDE EFFECTS OF ISONIAZID (INH)

- Acne
- Pellagra
- Neuropathy (with pyridoxine deficiency)
- Precipitation of epilepsy

ITRACONAZOLE: CONTRAINDICATIONS

- Astemizole and terfenadine = torsades de pointes
- All statins (i.e., simvastatin) = rhabdomyolysis, hepatotoxicity
- Alprazolam, midazolam, and triazolam = increased sedation
- Zafirkulast

SIDE EFFECTS OF KETOCONAZOLE

- Impotence
- Gynecomastia

TABLE 11–38
L-ASPARAGINASE[a]

Cutaneous Side Effects		Systemic Side Effects
Hypersensitivity reactions Urticarial (amyloidosis)	Itching + swelling of feet Toxic epidermal necrolysis	Anaphylaxis/hypotension/dyspnea Serum sickness

[a] Mechanism: Not cell cycle–specific, leukemia drug digests asparagines, starving leukemia tumor cells.

TABLE 11–39
LEUPROLIDE[a]

Cutaneous Side Effects		Systemic Side Effects
Drug-induced lupus	Flushing	Temporary worsening; hot flashes

[a] Mechanism: Potent GnRH analog; suppresses ovarian/testicular steroidogenesis (including androgens).

SIDE EFFECTS OF LITHIUM

- Linear IgA disease
- Exacerbates psoriasis, acne, Darier disease, dermatitis herpetiformis
- Gingival hyperplasia
- Ulcerations
- Acanthosis nigricans

MAST CELL DEGRANULATORS

A–	Anesthetics	Narcotics	Others	Cytokines
• Aspirin • Alcohol • Amphotericin B	• Decamethonium • Gallamine • Scopolamine • Tubocurarine • Quinine	• Codeine • Morphine	• Radiographic dyes • Reserpine • Polymyxin • Urticaceae (nettles) • Vancomycin • Benzoates	• IL-1

Mnemonic: PIANO

These mast cell degranulators cause major histamine release in patients with urticaria pigmentosa.

- Phenolphthalein
- Intravenous dye
- Anesthetics/aspirin
- Narcotics
- Opiates

TABLE 11–40
MECHLORETHAMINE (NITROGEN MUSTARD)[a]

Cutaneous Side Effects		Systemic Side Effects
Pruritus Urticaria	Allergic contact hypersensitivity Hyperpigmentation in occluded areas	Angioedema SCC/BCC

[a] Mechanism: Cross-links (alkylates) DNA, inhibiting DNA replication.

TABLE 11–41
MELPHALAN[a,b]

Cutaneous Side Effects		Systemic Side Effects
Hypersensitivity reactions Acral erythema	Nails: transverse white bands or longitudinal nail pigment bands	Bone marrow suppression Leukemia

[a] Used in the treatment of scleromyxedema and metastatic melanoma.
[b] Mechanism: Bifunctional alkylating agent (nitrogen mustard type).

TABLE 11–42
METHOTREXATE (MTX) PLUS ANALOGS: EDATRAXATE AND TRIMETREXATE

Mechanism	Inhibit dihydrofolate reductase, thus inhibiting DNA synthesis (purine). Inhibit thymidylate synthetase (pyrimidine).
Medications that raise MTX levels—and how	Salicylates, NSAIDs, sulfas—by displacing MTX from plasma proteins and lowering renal excretion. Dipyridamole and probenicid, by increasing the accumulation of MTX. Chloramphenicol, phenothiazines, phenytoin, and tetracycline, by displacing MTX from plasma proteins. Hypoalbuminemia increases MTX toxicity.
Medications that inhibit the folate pathway by increasing bone marrow suppression	Trimethoprim, sulfonamides, dapsone; these also inhibit dihydrofolate reductase.

TABLE 11–43
METHOTREXATE

Cutaneous Side Effects		Systemic Side Effects
Phototoxic	UV recall	Hepatotoxicity
Acral erythema	Nail pigmentation	Pulmonary fibrosis
Diffuse brownish pigmentation	Paronychia	Pneumonitis
Flag sign of hair hyper-/ hypopigmentation	Porphyria cutanea tarda	Lymphoma
Folliculitis/furnculosis/ acne exacerbation	Bullous pemphigoid (with dactinomycin)	Osteopathy
Ulceration over pressure areas	Cutaneous vasculitis	
Trimetrexate: flushing	Toxic epidermal necrolysis	
	Edetraxate: erythematous lesions on legs	

TABLE 11–44
6-MERCAPTOPURINE (6-MP)[a]

Cutaneous Side Effects		Systemic Side Effects
Photoonycholysis Vasculitis	Acral erythema	Bone marrow + liver toxicity

[a] Mechanism: Purine analog; inhibits DNA synthesis.

TABLE 11–45
MINOCYCLINE AND OTHER TETRACYCLINES

Mechanism	Bind 30S ribosomal unit inhibiting protein synthesis.
Drugs decrease absorption of tetracyclines (TCNs)	Calcium/cations: chelate tetracyclines. Cimetidine + $NaHCO_3$ induce pH-dependent inhibition of drug dissolution. Anticonvulsants decrease doxycycline levels.
TCNs cause effects on other drug levels	Digoxin, lithium, warfarin levels are increased. Insulin requirements are decreased.
Contraindications	Hepatic disease, renal failure (except doxycyline because of prolonged half-life. Can be given to children after age 8.

TABLE 11–46
MINOCYCLINE AND OTHER TETRACYCLINES

Cutaneous Side Effects		Systemic Side Effects
Photosensitivity Lupus-like rash, p-ANCA positive Pigmentation	Onycholysis Sweet syndrome	Pseudotumor cerebri Autoimmune hepatitis Pneumonitis Serum sickness

PIGMENTATION EFFECTS OF TETRACYCLINES[a]

Clinical/Location	Perls/Prussian Blue	Fontana-Masson
Blue acne scars	+	–
Blue shins	+	+
Photodistributed muddy brown	–	+

[a] The use of tetracyclines should be avoided in sclerotherapy patients because of resulting pigmentation.

TABLE 11–47
MITHRAMYCIN/PLICAMYCIN[a]

Cutaneous Side Effects		Systemic Side Effects
Intense facial erythema/ edema leading to patchy facial pigmentation + coarse facial features	Toxic epidermal necrolysis	Severe thrombocytopenia

[a] Mechanism: Complexes with DNA, which inhibits RNA synthesis.

TABLE 11–48
MITOMYCIN C[a, b]

Cutaneous Side Effects		Systemic Side Effects
Nails: purple pigmented bands	Hyperpigmentation	Anaphylaxis/angioedema
Exfoliation	Phototoxic effects	Hemolytic-uremic syndrome
Acral erythema	Pruritic vesicles: face, chest, palms, soles	
Allergic contact dermatitis (intravesical mitomycin)	Pityriasis rosea	

[a] Mechanism: Inhibits DNA synthesis by cross-linking with guanine and cytosine.
[b] Use DMSO for extravasation.

TABLE 11–49
MITOTANE[a]

Cutaneous Side Effects	Systemic Side Effects
Acral erythema	Severe adrenal suppression

[a] Mechanism: Adrenal cytotoxic agent; modifies peripheral steroid metabolism to suppress adrenal function.

TABLE 11–50
MITOXANTRONE[a]

Cutaneous Side Effects		Systemic Side Effects
Vasculitis	Hyperpigmenation: face, dorsal hands, nails	Anaphylaxis
Urticaria/pruritus	Neutrophilic eccrine hidradenitis	Angioedema

[a] Mechanism: Not cell cycle–specific; DNA-reactive agent (miscellaneous chemo).

TABLE 11–51
MYCOPHENOLATE MOFETIL/CELLCEPT[a,b]

Cutaneous Side Effects	Systemic Side Effects	
Increased risk of herpes zoster	Gastrointestinal + genitourinary side effects CMV viremia	Neutropenia/leukopenia Mild neurologic effects

[a] Mechanism: Inhibits purine synthesis via inhibition of inosine monophosphate dehydrogenase in the de novo purine biosynthesis pathway through inhibition of proliferating B and T cells (non-bone marrow).
[b] Contraindication: Cholestyramine.

CROSS REACTIONS OF NEOMYCIN

- Bacitracin
- Gentamicin[a]
- Tobramycin
- Streptomycin
- Paromomycin
- Butirosin

[a] All gentamicin topicals can be nephrotoxic.

TABLE 11–52
PACLITAXEL (TAXOL)[a]

Cutaneous Side Effects		Systemic Side Effects
Hypersensitivity reactions (2–4%) Urticaria	Flushing + acral erythema Bullous fixed drug reaction	Dyspnea + hypotension Anaphylaxis/angioedema

[a] Mechanism: Inhibits proper microtubule function.

SIDE EFFECTS OF PENTAMIDINE

- Nephrotoxic
- Cardiac effects
- Pancreatitis
- Sterile intramuscular abscesses

PENTAVALENT ANTIMONY

Monitor ECG during administration.

TABLE 11–53
PENTOSTATIN[a]

Cutaneous Side Effects	Systemic Side Effects	
Inflammation of actinic keratoses	Renal, liver, CNS toxicity	Fatal pulmonary toxicity with fludarabine

[a] Mechanism: Inhibits adenosine deaminase because it blocks DNA synthesis (via RNA reductase). Also, to lesser degree, inhibits RNA synthesis and DNA repair.

SIDE EFFECTS OF PERIACTIN

Used in cold urticaria.

- Increased appetite and weight gain
- Growth retardation

TABLE 11–54
PHENYTOIN: CUTANEOUS SIDE EFFECTS[a]

Acneiform rash	Pseudolymphoma
Gingival hyperplasia	Vasculitis
Lupus-like symptoms	Chloasma
Dermatomyositis-like eruption, then depigmentation	Pellagra

[a] Hypersensitivity syndrome due to deficiency of epoxide hydroxylase.

SIDE EFFECTS OF PIMOZIDE

- QT prolongation (most common)
- Cardiomyopathy
- Tardive dyskinesias (dose related)

SIDE EFFECTS OF PODOPHYLLIN

Used to treat oral hairy leukoplakiaanogenital warts.

- Binds tubulin and stops mitosis, arrests metaphase
- "Starburst" keratinocytes arrested in metaphase on pathology

TABLE 11–55
PROCARBAZINE[a]

Cutaneous Side Effects		Systemic Side Effects
Diffuse melanosis	Phototoxicity	CNS toxicity
Toxic epidermal necrolysis	Flushing	Bone marrow suppression
Fixed drug reaction		

[a] Mechanism: Inhibits t-RNA formation, thus inhibiting protein synthesis and subsequently DNA/RNA synthesis.

QUINOLONES

- Act on DNA gyrase (DNA topoisomerase II).
- Contraindicated in children because of arthropathy.

TABLE 11–56
RETINOIDS AND RECEPTORS[a,b]

Retinoid	Half-Life	Receptor Binding	Odd Side Effects to Know	
Tretinoin	1 h	All RARs		
Adapalene	1 h	RAR-β and γ (not α)		
Tazarotene	1 h	RAR-β and γ (not α)		
Panretin		RARs + RXRα + CRABPs		
Bexarotene	7–9 h	Only RXR-α	Hypothyroidism	Gemfibrozil raises level of drug
Isotretinoin	10–20 h	All RARs		
Acitretin	50 h	All RARs	Pyogenic granuloma Inflammatory bowel disease flare	Agranulocytosis + leukopenia Need oral contraceptives until 3 years after last dose
Etretinate	80–160 days	All RARs		

[a] RARs (α, β, γ): skin, γ most common.
[b] RXRs: basal and follicular epithelium.

TABLE 11–57
RIFAMPIN[a,b]

Cutaneous Side Effects		Systemic Side Effects
Orange secretions ("red man")	Pemphigoid-like reaction	P450 inducer
Pruritus/urticaria	Acneiform reaction	Hypersensitivity reactions
Exfoliation	Conjunctivitis	GI, hepatic, renal, CNS toxicity
		Acute hemolytic anemia

[a] Inhibits RNA polymerase.
[b] Contraindications: Combined with INH, increases hepatotoxicity; combined with enalapril, may increase blood pressure.

TABLE 11–58
RITUXIMAB[a]

Uses	Systemic Side Effects	
B-cell lymphoma	Infusion-related fever/chills/ headache	Bronchospasm, hypotension

[a] Mechanism: Chimeric murine/human monoclonal antibody against CD-20.

SIDE EFFECT OF ROQUINEMEX

Eccrine sweat gland necrosis.

SIDE EFFECTS OF SALICYLIC ACID

Tinnitus, confusion, psychosis, refractory hypoglycemia (especially in diabetics and patients with chronic renal failure).

SIDE EFFECTS OF SATURATED POTASSIUM IODIDE (SSKI)

- Exacerbates dermatitis herpetiformis, pyoderma gangrenosum, pustular psoriasis (neutrophilic dermatoses)
- Iodaderma
- Acne
- Erythema nodosum
- Erythema multiforme

TABLE 11–59
SURAMIN[a]

Cutaneous Side Effects (Systemic Unknown)	
Acral erythema + flushing	UV recall
Keratotic papules	Toxic epidermal necrolysis

[a] Mechanism: Unknown.

TABLE 11–60
SYSTEMIC SIDE EFFECTS OF TACROLIMUS/PIMECROLIMUS[a,b]

Renal impairment	Insomnia	Hyperglycemia
Hypertension	↑K, ↓Mg	

[a] Mechanism: Binds to calcineurin via FKBP-12, stopping NFAT dephosphorylation, which blocks IL-2 trancription.
[b] Netherton syndrome.

TABLE 11–61
TAMOXIFEN[a]

Cutaneous Side Effects		Systemic Side Effects
Dermatomyositis-like eruption	Flushing	Deep venous thrombosis
Hair color change	Vasculitis	Pulmonary embolism
Hirsutism		Hepatotoxicity
		Serum sickness

[a] Mechanism: Nonsteroidal antiestrogen; competes with estrogen binding in target tissues (i.e., breast).

TABLE 11–62
THALIDOMIDE[a]

Cutaneous Side Effects	Systemic Side Effects	
Xerostomia	Teratogenicity: phocomelia	Peripheral neuropathy (sensory)
Brittle fingernails	Hypothyroidism	
Red palms	Leukopenia	Drowsiness (sedative)
	Increased appetite	Constipation
	Irregular menses	Decreased libido

[a] Proposed mechanism: anti-TNF-α.

TABLE 11–63
6-THIOGUANINE[a]

Cutaneous Side Effects		Systemic Side Effects
Inflammation of actinic keratoses	Phototoxicity	Bone marrow + liver toxicity

[a] Mechanism: Purine analog; inhibits DNA synthesis.

TABLE 11–64
CUTANEOUS SIDE EFFECTS OF TEGAFUR

Hyperpigmentation: 33% patients develop discrete 0.5-cm dark macules on palms, soles, nails, penis, and lips	Acral erythema Lichenoid eruption	Dermatomyositis + lupus-like reaction Photoallergy and phototoxicity

TABLE 11–65
THIOTEPA (TRIETHYLENETHIOPHOSPHORAMIDE)[a]

Cutaneous Side Effects		Systemic Side Effects
Hyperpigmentation: occluded sites (ECG pads) due to increased levels in sweat, which is toxic to melanocytes	Leukoderma (eyelashes and eyelids after topical use)	Bone marrow toxicity Leukemia

[a] Mechanism: Alkylates guanine bases disrupting DNA bonds.

TABLE 11–66
UV-PHOTOPROTECTIVE SYSTEMIC AGENTS

Agent	Spectrum
α-Tocopherol	UVB
Ascorbic acid	UVB
β-Carotene (can cause yellow-orange palms and soles)	Visible
Antimalarials	UVB/UVA
Polypodium leukotomus	UVA + antioxidant

TABLE 11–67
VINCA ALKALOIDS (VINBLASTINE/VINCRISTINE/VINORELBINE)[a,b]

Cutaneous Side Effects		Systemic Side Effects
Heat with infiltration; cold application leads to ulcerations	Phototoxicity	Leukopenia
Raynaud phenomenon	Inflammation of actinic keratoses	Neutropenia
Flare of dermatitis herpetiformis with cytoxan + doxorubicin	Leukonychia (vincristine)	Use hyaluronic acid to treat extravasation
Supravenous hyperpigmentation (vinorelbine)	Acral erythema	
	Acne	

[a]Mechanism: Interferes with amino acid metabolic pathways, leading to metaphase arrest.
[b]Intralesional vinblastine used to treat localized Kaposi sarcoma.

SECTION II

QUICK GUIDE TO MEDICATION REACTIONS

ACANTHOLYSIS IN VITRO

- Penicillamine
- Captopril
- Piroxicam

ACANTHOSIS NIGRICANS

- OCPs
- Niacin
- Diethylstilbestrol
- Azathioprine
- Gemfibrozil
- Lithium
- Mechlorethamine
- Thioridazine
- Heroin

DIFFERENTIAL DIAGNOSIS OF DRUG-INDUCED ACNE

Chemotherapeutic Agents

- Lithium
- Bromides/iodides
- INH
- Antimalarials
- ACTH
- Steroids
- Phenytoin
- Penicillins
- Chloral hydrate
- Scopolamine
- Dactinomycin
- Vinblastine

DIFFERENTIAL DIAGNOSIS OF ACRAL ERYTHEMA

Chemotherapy-induced, usually dose-related:

- Cytarabine (Ara-C)
- Daunorubicin/idarubicin
- Lomustine
- Mitotane
- Doxorubicin
- Docetaxel
- Melphalan
- Paclitaxel
- 5-FU
- Doxifluridine
- Mercaptopurine
- Suramin
- Cisplatin
- Etoposide
- Methotrexate
- Tegafur
- Cyclophosphamide
- Hydroxyurea
- Mitomycin
- Vincristine

ACUTE GENERALIZED EXANTHEMATOUS PUSTULOSIS (AGEP)

- β-Lactams
- Macrolides
- Lamisil (terbinafine)

AMPICILLIN

With the following, can lead to rash:

- Epstein-Barr virus (mono) (80% of patients)
- Cytomegalovirus
- Allopurinol
- Chronic lymphocytic leukemia

ANGIOEDEMA

Can be caused by ACE inhibitors

INDUCERS OF BULLOUS PEMPHIGOID

- Furosemide
- Methotrexate and dactinomycin
- Potassium-sparing diuretics
- Ampicillin
- Chlorpromazine

INDUCERS OF CICATRICIAL PEMPHIGOID

- Penicillamine
- Clonidine
- Practolol
- Eye topicals (unilateral)

DRUGS THAT EXACERBATE DERMATITIS HERPETIFORMIS

Chemotherapeutic Agents

- NSAIDs/ASA
- SSKI/iodine
- IFN-α
- Pentoxifylline
- Amitriptyline
- Lithium
- OCPs
- Levothyroxine
- Cyclophosphamide
- Vincristine
- Doxorubicin

DIFFERENTIAL DIAGNOSIS OF DERMATOMYOSITIS-LIKE REACTION

Chemotherapeutic Agents

- Penicillamine
- Carbamazepine
- Practolol
- Phenytoin
- NSAIDs (phenylbutazone)
- Pravastatin
- BCG vaccine
- Hydroxyurea
- Tamoxifen
- Tegafur

DISULFURAM-LIKE REACTION (ANTABUSE)

- Cefotetan
- Metronidazole

CAUSES OF ERYTHEMA ANNULARE CENTRIFIGUM

- Gold
- Thiazides
- Antimalarials
- Penicillin
- NSAIDs
- Aldactone

CAUSES OF ERYTHEMA MULTIFORME MAJOR

1. Trimethoprim-sulfamethoxazole (Bactrim)
2. Dilantin (most common in children)
3. Carbamazepine
4. Phenobarbital
5. Allopurinol

CAUSES OF FIXED DRUG REACTIONS

Chemotherapeutic Agents

- Bactrim
- ASA
- Phenolphthalein
- Barbiturates
- OCPs
- Phenylbutazone
- NSAIDs
- Phenytoin
- Tetracyclines
- Foscarnet
- Metronidazole
- Dacarbazine
- Hydroxyurea
- Paclitaxel (bullous fixed drug)
- Procarbazine

CAUSES OF GINGIVAL HYPERPLASIA

- Calcium channel blockers
- Phenytoin/anticonvulsants
- OCPs/estrogen
- Cyclosporine
- Erythromycin
- Sertraline (Zoloft)
- Lithium
- Ketoconazole
- Ethosuximide

CAUSES OF HAIR COLOR CHANGE

- Cyclophosphamide: light red to black
- Cisplatin
- Methotrexate: flag sign
- Bleomycin/doxorubicin/vincristine: black to red

CAUSES OF HYPERPIGMENTATION (PECULIAR TYPES)

Flagellate	Under Occlusion (ECG Pads)	Sites of Pressure	Blue-Gray Facial
• Bleomycin[a] • Fluorouracil	• Carmustine • Mechlorethamine • Ifosfamide • Thiotepa • Docetaxel • Brequinar	Cisplatin Bleomycin Hydroxyurea	• Chlorpromazine (Fontana-Masson +) • Amiodarone (PAS+) • Minocycline • Ochronosis • Argyria • Chrysiasis
Supravenous Serpentine			
• Fluorouracil • Fotemustine • Vinorelbine • Dactinomycin	• Etoposide/carboplatin + cytoxan or ifosfamide		• Diltiazem • Imipramine • Doxorubicin • Mercury (eyelids, nasolabial fold, neck)

[a]Flagellate erythema is associated with dermatomyositis and correlates with disease activity.

TABLE 11–68
HYPERPIGMENTATION (OTHER TYPES)

Drug	Type of Pigmentation
Busulfan	"Dusky" bronze/brown, generalized
Cyclophosphamide	Patchy or generalized, irreversible on teeth
Ifosfamide	Flexural areas, dorsal hands/feet, scrotum, trunk
Cisplatin	70% of patients with patchy type
Fluorouracil	Sun-exposed tanning, widespread reticulate, or palms/soles
Tegafur	One-third with macules on palms/soles/lips/penis
Methotrexate	Generalized brownish
Bleomycin	Patchy and in new striae
Dactinomycin	Diffuse melanosis
Daunorubicin	Sun-exposed and polycyclic scalp
Doxorubicin	Generalized
Plicamycin/ mithramycin	Patchy pigmentation on face after intense facial eruption
Mitoxantrone	Face and dorsal hands
Hydroxyurea	Generalized
Procarbazine	Diffuse melanosis
Minocycline	Patchy blue or muddy brown
Perfloxacin	Bluish
Antimalarials	Yellow skin/conjunctivae; blue-black cartilage/palate/nail bed
Clofazimine	Red-brown in lesions, lipofuscin-positive
Antipsychotics	Photo-induced, generalized

CAUSES OF HYPERTRICHOSIS

- Cyclosporine
- Phenytoin
- Diazoxide
- Steroids
- Aldactone
- Phenothiazines
- Minoxidil
- Hunter-Hurler syndrome

CAUSES OF ICHTHYOSIS (ACQUIRED)

- Nicotinic acid
- Triparanol
- Butyrophenones (antipsychotics)
- Nafodine (estrogen antagonist)
- Dixyramine (major tranquilizer)

INFLAMMATION OF LESIONS

Actinic Keratoses	Seborrheic Keratoses	Squamous Cell Carcinoma
• Docetaxel • Doxorubicin • Fluorouracil • Pentostatin • Dactinomycin • Vincristine • Dacarbazine • Cytarabine • 6-Thioguanine • Cisplatin	• Cytarabine	• Fludarabine

CAUSES OF LEUKOCYTOCLASTIC VASCULITIS

- Insulin
- Penicillin
- Sulfonamides
- Hydantoins
- Streptomycin
- β Blockers
- Aminosalicylic acid
- Thiazides
- Phenothiazines
- Phenylbutazone
- Quinine
- Streptokinase
- Tamoxifen
- Influenza vaccine
- Oral contraceptives
- Propylthiouracil
- Iodides

CAUSES OF LEUKODERMA

- Thiotepa
- Benzoquinone
- Phenytoin
- Phenol

LICHENOID DRUG ERUPTIONS

β Blockers
Antimalarials
Penicillamine
ACE inhibitors
Calcium channel blockers
NSAIDs
Allopurinol
Dapsone
Phenytoin
Aldactone
Simvastatin
Metformin
Sulfasalazine
Methamphetamines
Tegafur
Chlorpropamide
Tolazamide
Torsemide
Meprobamate
Chenodeoxycholic acid
Cycloserine
Cyanide
Ribavirin plus IFN-α

Photodistributed	Pemphigoid	Ulcerative	Oral Lichen Planus Lesions
Quinine	Captopril	Hydroxyurea	Antihypertensives
Quinidine	Cinnarizine	Methyldopa	NSAIDs
Thiazides		Propanolol	Contact allergens
Furosemide	**Bullous**	Lithium	Dental fillings (amalgam)
Diazoxide	Labetalol		Dental implants
Tetracyclines		**Contact Dermatitis**	
Chlorpromazine	**Pigmentosus**	Phenylenediamines	
Carbamazepine	Gold (also contact dermatitis)	Aminoglycosides	
		Musk ambrette	
		Nickel	

LINEAR IgA DISEASE: DRUG ASSOCIATIONS

- Vancomycin
- Diclofenac
- Bactrim
- Phenytoin
- ACE inhibitors
- Lithium
- Captopril
- Somatostatin
- Glyburide
- Amiodarone
- PCN
- PUVA
- Furosemide
- Rifampin
- Oxaprozin
- IL-2
- IFN-γ
- IFN-α

DIFFERENTIAL DIAGNOSIS OF NAIL PIGMENTATION

Blue Discoloration		Brown Discoloration
Argyria	Phenolphthalein	Busulfan
AZT (zidovudine)	Chemotherapy	
Wilson disease	Hemoglobin M	

LUPUS: DRUG-INDUCED

Antihistone-positive *except* penicillamine, which is anti-dsDNA-positive; minocycline is p-ANCA-positive.

-INE	-IDE	Other	Chemo
Chlorpromazine	Isoniazid	Methyldopa	DES
Hydralazine	Procainamide	Phenytoin	Hydroxyurea
Penicillamine	Sulfonamide	Minocycline	Tegafur
Quinidine	Aminoglutethimide		
Terbinafine	Leuprolide		

DIFFERENTIAL DIAGNOSIS OF NAIL PIGMENTATION DUE TO MEDICATIONS

Blue			Leukonychia
Disease	Meds	Chemo	
			Aminoglutethimide
Hemochromatosis	Antimalarials	Doxorubicin	Cisplatin
Wilson disease	Minocin	Fluorouracil (nail bed)	Cytarabine (transverse bands)
Ochronosis/ Alkaptonuria	Silver nitrate		Daunorubicin
	AZT (nail bed)		Melphalan (transverse bands)
			Vincristine
Banding	**Purple**	**Brown**	
Bleomycin	Mitomycin (bands)	Busulfan	
Doxorubicin (horizontal + longitudinal)		Daunorubicin (horizontal bands)	
Fluorouracil		Hydroxyurea	
Hydroxyurea (longitudinal and transverse bands)			
Melphalan (longitudinal bands)			

CAUSES OF NEUTROPHILIC ECCRINE HIDRADENITIS

- Bleomycin
- Chlorambucil
- Cyclophosphamide
- Cytarabine
- Doxorubicin
- Lomustine
- Mitoxantrone

OCTREOTIDE

- Used intravenously with streptozocin for necrolytic migratory erythema to control pancreatic effects
- Used to treat carcinoid syndrome

CAUSES OF PELLAGRA

- Isoniazid
- Carcinoid syndrome
- Imuran
- Mercaptopurine
- 5-Fluorouracil
- Hydantoins/phenytoin
- Phenobarbital
- Pyrazinamide

PEMPHIGUS INDUCERS

Mnemonic: "PCP" = penicillamine, captopril, penicillins

- Rifampin
- Enalapril
- Pyrazolone
- Thiopronine
- Drugs with negatively charged domains (i.e., sulfhydryl groups)

PENICILLAMINE-INDUCED DERMATOSES

Bullous	Collagen/Elastin	Other
Pemphigus	Elastosis perforans serpiginosa	Yellow nail syndrome
Bullous and cicatrical pemphigoid	Pseudoxanthoma elasticum	Lichenoid drug reaction
Epidermolysis bullosa acquisita	Cutis laxa	Pityriasis rosea-like eruption
	Anetoderma	Lichen planus
	Subacute cutaneous lupus	Myasthenia syndrome
	Systemic lupus	Nephrotic syndrome
		Loss of taste
		Transient cutis laxa in baby whose mother received penicillamine

PHOTOONYCHOLYSIS

- Tetracycline
- 8-Methoxypsoralens
- Mercaptopurine
- OCPs
- Chloramphenicol
- Quinolones
- Benoxaprofen
- Quinine

DRUGS CAUSING PHOTOALLERGY REACTIONS

Photosensitizers	Sunscreens	Other
6-Methylcoumarin Salicylanilide Chlorothiazide (highest incidence)	PABA Benzophenones	Musk ambrette Benzocaine Chlorpromazine Neomycin NSAIDS • Sulfonamides

Phototoxic Drugs	Chemotherapeutic Drugs		
Amiodarone			
• Chlorpromazine	Brequinar	Dacarbazine	Dactinomycin
Fluoroquinolones: nalidixic acid, ciprofloxacin	Doxorubicin	Fluorouracil	Hydroxyurea
Griseofulvin	Methotrexate	Mitomycin C	Procarbazine
Tetracyclines: demeclocycline > doxycycline	Tegafur	Thioguanine	Vinblastine
NSAIDS: piroxicam, benoxaprofen (most phototoxic)			
Ibuprofen least phototoxic (does not absorb >310 nm)			

TABLE 11–69
PHOTOTOXIC VS. PHOTOALLERGIC

Characteristics	Phototoxic	Photoallergic
Appearance	Sunburn	Eczematous
Action spectrum	UVA + UVB	UVA
Erythema annulare centrifugum	Direct cell damage	Delayed-type hypersensitivity
Reaction to first exposure	Yes	No
Timing	Rapid	Delayed
Antigen concentration	High	Low
Pathology	Basal degeneration	Acute spongiotic dermatitis

PITYRIASIS ROSEA-LIKE DRUG ERUPTIONS

Mnemonic: "BCC GIMP"

Barbiturates
Captopril
Clonidine
Gold
Isotretinoin
Metronidazole/mitomycin C
Penicillamine

PORPHYRIAS (CHEMOTHERAPY-INDUCED)

Porphyria Cutanea Tarda	Acute Intermittent Porphyria	Pseudoporphyria
Busulfan Cyclophosphamide Diethylstilbestrol Methotrexate	Chlorambucil Cyclophosphamide	• Cisplatin

VARIEGATE DRUG-INDUCED PORPHYRIA

Mnemonic: "Begs For Alcohol or Safe"

Barbiturates
Estrogen
Griseofulvin
Sulfonamides
Alcohol

Sulfas, sedatives, sex, steroids
Anticonvulsants/alcohol Fungicides [griseofulvin linked to hereditary coporphyria (HCP)]
Ergotamines

DRUGS CAUSING PSEUDOPORPHYRIA

Mnemonic: "All dead fetuses need no pyridoxine or tetracycline."

- Amiodarone
- Dapsone
- Furosemide
- Nalidixic acid
- NSAIDS (Naproxen)
- Pyridoxine
- Tetracycline (high dose)
- UVA high dose
- CRF on hemodialysis (Bullous dermatosis of HD)

PSORALENS

8-Methoxypsoralens: dose at 0.6 mg/kg; photosensitivity lasts 8 h.

DRUGS EXACERBATING PSORIASIS

- β Blockers
- Ca^{2+} channel blockers
- Systemic steroids
- Gemfibrozil
- Terbinafine
- Captopril
- Alcohol
- Lithium
- Antimalarials
- Glyburide
- Inteferon (IFN) α/β
- GM-CSF
- IL-2
- Oral contraceptives
- NSAIDs
- Isoniazid
- Penicillamine
- SSKI (pustular)
- Aminoglutethimide

DRUGS CAUSING RAYNAUD PHENOMENON

- β Blockers
- IFN-α
- Aldactone
- Azathioprine
- Amphetamines
- Bromocriptine
- Clonidine

Chemotherapeutic Drugs
- Bleomycin
- Cisplatin
- Vinblastine/vincristine

DRUGS CAUSING RENAL NECROSIS

- Sulfapyridine
- Salicylic acid

DRUGS CAUSING SCOTOMA (Visual Field Defect)

- Hydroxychloroquine
- Chloroquine
- Ethambutol
- Antimalarials

DRUGS CAUSING SERUM SICKNESS

- Cefaclor
- Minocycline
- Thiazides
- Oral contraceptives
- PCNs
- Hydantoins
- Sulfas
- Vaccines
- ASA
- Streptokinase
- Tamoxifen

DRUGS CAUSING SWEET SYNDROME

- Minocycline
- Trimethoprim-sulfamethoxazole
- Glucagon
- G-CSF
- Cytarabine
- BCG and pneumococcal vaccines

DRUGS CAUSING SUBACUTE CUTANEOUS LUPUS

- Thiazides
- Aldactone
- Piroxicam
- Naproxen
- Penicillamine
- Gold
- Griseofulvin
- Sulfonylureas
- Procainamide
- Oxyprenolol
- Phenothiazine

ACE Inhibitors
- Captopril

Calcium Channel Blockers
- Diltiazem
- Verapamil
- Nifedipine

β Blockers

DRUGS CAUSING TOXIC EPIDERMAL NECROLYSIS

- Antibiotics (sulfonamides > penicillins, cephalosporins, quinolones)
- Anticonvulsants
- NSAIDs (piroxicam)
- Allopurinol
- Steroids

Reactions more common in HIV-positive patients

Chemotherapeutic Drugs

- Bleomycin
- Chlorambucil
- Cytarabine
- Doxorubicin
- 5-FU
- L-asparaginase
- MTX
- Plicamycin/ mithramycin
- Procarbazine
- Suramin

CAUSES OF ACQUIRED TRICHOMEGALY (LONGER EYELASHES)

- HIV disease
- IFN-α_{2A} therapy (for non-Hodgkin lymphoma)
- Cyclosporine
- Chronic illness
- Kala-azar (Pitalnga's sign)
- Malnutrition

DRUGS CAUSING UV RECALL

- Etoposide
- Cyclophosphamide
- Methotrexate
- Fluorouracil
- Suramin

Vasculitis (Leukocytoclastic)

- Insulin
- Penicillin
- Sulfonamides
- Hydantoins
- Streptomycin
- Propylthiouracil
- β Blockers
- Aminosalicylic acid
- Thiazides
- Phenothiazines
- Phenylbutazone
- Quinine
- Streptokinase
- Iodides (pustular)
- Influenza vaccine
- Oral contraceptives

Chemotherapeutic Drugs

- Busulfan
- Cyclophosphamide
- Cytarabine
- Hydroxyurea
- Levamisole
- Hexamethylene bisacetamide (HMBA)
- 6-Mercaptopurine
- Methotrexate
- Mitoxantrone
- Tamoxifen

CHAPTER 12

HIGH-YIELD FACTOIDS

ASSOCIATIONS WITH ARSENIC

- Superficial BCCs
- Mees lines (nail plate)
- Anemia
- Pancytopenia
- Hyperpigmented patches
- Fowler solution
- Pressure-treated wood that is burned
- Actinic keratoses
- Neuropathy
- RBC "cloverleaf nucleus"
- Metallic breath odor
- Hepatic angiosarcoma
- Contaminated well water
- Merkel cell carcinoma, genitourinary and pulmonary carcinoma

BLOOD GROUP A

Increased susceptibility to superficial fungal infections

BLUE SCLERAE

- Ochronosis/alkaptonuria
- Argyria
- Nevus of Ota
- Ehlers-Danlos syndrome
- Incontinentia pigmenti
- Osteogenesis imperfecta
- Quinacrine

DERMOSCOPY/EPILUMINESCENCE MICROSCOPY (ELM)

- Maple leaf = pigmented BCC
- Pseudohorn cyst = SK
- Streaking and blue veil = Melanoma
- Lagoons = vascular dilatation (cherry angiomas)
- Dots = SK
- Slate blue = blue nevus

DIFFERENTIAL DIAGNOSIS OF ECZEMA HERPETICUM

Also known as Kaposi varicelliform eruption

Dermatitis	Acantholytic	Keratin Disorders	Cancer	Infectious
Atopic dermatitis	Pemphigus	Ichthyosis vulgaris	CTCL	Rubeola
Wiskott-Aldrich syndrome	Darier syndrome	EHK	Sézary syndrome	
Neurodermatitis	Hailey-Hailey syndrome			
Seborrheic dermatitis				

DIFFERENTIAL DIAGNOSIS OF HERTOGH[a] SIGN (Lateral Eyebrow Hair Loss)

Mnemonic: STEAL U-Haul

- Syphilis
- Trichotillomania
- Ectodermal dysplasia
- Alopecia areata/mucinosa
- Leprosy
- Ulerythema ophryogenes
- Hypothyroidism

[a] Noonan's syndrome and Rubinstein-Taybi syndrome

TABLE 12–1
HYPERPIGMENTATION AND HYPOPIGMENTATION: FOCAL AND DIFFUSE

Entity	Number of Melanocytes	Melanosomes/Activity
Lentigines (solar, PUVA)	↑	Normal + macromelanosomes
Melasma	↑	Normal
Delayed tanning (UVB)	↑	Normal
Café-au-lait macules (McCune-Albright)	↑	Macromelanosomes (NF-1)
Nevus spilus	↑	Macromelanosomes
Ephiledes	Normal	↑
Becker nevus	Normal	↑
Labial melanotic macule	Normal	↑
Dowling-Degos disease	Normal	↑
Cirrhosis hyperpigmentation	Normal	↑ Melanin in giant melanosomes
Piebaldism	None	
Pityriasis alba	↓	Normal
Tuberous sclerosis	↓	↓ Melanosome size, ↓ melanin synthesis
Cross syndrome	↓	Hair bulb incubation test: weak
Nevus anemicus	Normal	↑Sensitivity of vessels to catecholamines; not dermatographic; relieve with sympathetic blockade
Menkes kinky hair	Normal	↓ Tyrosinase activity
Tinea versicolor	Normal	↓ Tyrosinase activity
Nevus depigmentosus	Normal	Defect in melanosome transfer
Griscelli syndrome	Normal	Defect in melanosome transfer; giant melanosomes in hair
Albinism	Normal	↓ Melanin synthesis

Note: ACTH is analogous to alpha-MSH.

DIFFERENTIAL DIAGNOSIS OF KOEBNERIZATION

- Vitiligo
- Lichen planus
- Erythema multiforme
- Psoriasis
- Warts
- Sweet syndrome
- Molluscum contagiosum
- Darier's
- Perforating disorders

DIFFERENTIAL DIAGNOSIS OF LEONINE FACIES

- CTCL
- Leprosy (lepromatous)
- Leishmaniasis
- Sarcoid
- Multiple trichoepitheliomas
- Actinic reticuloid
- Papular mucinosis/scleromyxedema
- Amyloidosis

DIFFERENTIAL DIAGNOSIS OF LETHAL MIDLINE GRANULOMA

- Lymphoma (NHL) (EBV and HTLV-1 associations)
- Angiocentric T-cell lymphoma
- Wegener granulomatosis

DIFFERENTIAL DIAGNOSIS OF LIVEDO RETICULARIS

- Leukocytoclastic vasculitis
- Diabetes
- Tuberculosis
- Polycythemia vera
- Pheochromocytoma
- Cryoglobulins (early)
- Polyarteritis nodosa
- Scleroderma
- Syphilis
- Anticardiolipin antibody
- Drug-induced (amantadine)
- Protein C deficiency
- Systemic lupus
- Rheumatoid arthritis
- Rheumatic fever
- Oxalate deposits
- Congenital (cutis marmorata)
- Homocystinuria

MALAKOPLAKIA

- Michaelis-Gutman bodies
- von-Hansemann cells
- *Escherichia coli* most common etiology
- Most common location: urinary tract
- Treat with quinolones, trimethoprim-sulfamethoxazole, penicillin, clofazimine, bethanecol, ascorbic acid

DIFFERENTIAL DIAGNOSIS OF MARFANOID HABITUS

- Ehlers-Danlos syndrome type VI
- Homocystinuria
- Multiple endocrine neoplasia type 2B (MEN 2B)
- Marfan syndrome
- Basal cell nevus syndrome (Gorlin syndrome)

MELANOSOMES: STAGES

- I, II: tyrosinase-negative
- III, IV: tyrosinase-positive
- Eumelanin: darker, need tyrosinase-related protein-2 (TRP-2)
- Pheomelanin: lighter (contains cysteine)

DIFFERENTIAL DIAGNOSIS OF MIDLINE FACIAL NODULE

- Dermoid cyst
- Hemangioma
- Rhabdomyosarcoma
- Epidermoid cyst
- Nasolacrimal duct cyst
- Meningocele
- Nasal glioma—does not transilluminate or enlarge with crying
- Encephalocele—may also be intracranial

DIFFERENTIAL DIAGNOSIS OF PALMAR PITS

- Punctate keratoderma in blacks
- Punctate porokeratosis
- Pitted keratolysis (usually feet)
- Arsenical keratoses
- Basal cell nevus syndrome
- Ectodermal dysplasia
- Darier disease
- Eccrine duct nevus

TABLE 12–2
SIGNS OF PANCREATITIS

Sign	Clinical Manifestations
Cullen	Periumbilical hematoma
Grey-Turner	Hematoma on flanks and/or groin
Walzel	Livedo reticularis on flank

DIFFERENTIAL DIAGNOSIS OF PAPULOSQUAMOUS ERUPTIONS

- Psoriasis
- Seborrheic dermatitis
- Atopic dermatitis
- Cutaneous T-cell lymphoma (CTCL)/parapsoriasis
- Pityriasis rubra pilaris
- Pityriasis lichenoides et varioliformis acuta (PLEVA)/Pityriasis lichenoides chronica (PLC)
- Tinea versicolor
- Lichen simplex chronicus
- Guttate psoriasis
- Reiter syndrome
- Lichen planus
- Pityriasis rosea

DIFFERENTIAL DIAGNOSIS OF ANNULAR PAPULOSQUAMOUS ERUPTIONS

- Granuloma annulare
- Pityriasis rosea
- Tinea corporis
- SCLE
- Annular psoriasis
- Annular lichen planus
- Discoid lupus
- Erythema annulare centrifugum

PARAPROTEINEMIAS ASSOCIATED WITH SKIN CHANGES

IgG Gammopathy (most common: λ vs. κ)

- Plasmacytoma/myeloma (κ)
- Amyloid (λ = two-thirds of patients)
- POEMS (λ)
- Scleromyxedema/lichen myxedematosus (λ)
- Scleredema (not associated with upper respiratory infection or diabetes) (κ)
- Necrobiotic xanthogranuloma (κ) (80% of patients)
- Normolipemic plane xanthomas (λ)

Rare

- Angioimmunoblastic lymphadenopathy
- Eosinophilic fasciitis
- Rosai-Dorfman disease (90% of patients) (sinus histiocytosis with lymphadenopathy)
- Acquired angioedema I

IgA Monoclonal Gammopathy (SEP)

- PG (10% of patients)
- Sweet syndrome (4%)
- Erythema elevatum diutinum
- Subcorneal pustular dermatosis
- Primary cutaneous plasmacytoma (20% become myeloma)

IgM Gammopathy (most common = κ)

- Schnitzler syndrome = urticaria, bone pain, and hyperostosis
- Waldenstrom hyperglobulinemic purpura

Other

- Cryoglobulinemia (type 1 = monoclonal)
- 25% of cases of monoclonal gammopathy unknown significance (MGUS) become plasma cell dyscrasias
- Half-life IgG = 3 weeks, except IgG3 = 1 week

CLINICAL DIFFERENTIAL DIAGNOSIS OF PELLAGRA

Pellagra results from a deficiency of tryptophan or niacin.

- The four D's: diarrhea, dermatitis, dementia, death
- Alcoholism/anorexia

- Carcinoid
- Hartnup disease (also treat with nicotinamide)
- Isoniazid
- Phenytoin

CAUSES OF PERIORBITAL PAPULES

- Dermatosis papulosa nigra
- Syringomas
- Trichoepitheliomas
- Xanthelasma
- Sarcoidosis
- Acne agminata
- Amyloid
- Desmoid tumor
- Hidrocystoma (epocrine = bluish, eccrine = small, shiny)

DIFFERENTIAL DIAGNOSIS OF PHOTOSENSITIVITY

- Phototoxic drug
- Solar urticaria
- Dermatomyositis
- PMLE
- Porphyrias: EPP, EP
- Xeroderma pigmentosum
- SLE
- Hydroa aestivale/vacciniforme
- Bloom/Cockayne/Rothmund-Thomson syndromes

DIFFERENTIAL DIAGNOSIS OF POIKILODERMA ATROPHICANS VASCULARE

Malignancy	CT Disease	Genodermatoses	Infectious
MF/parapsoriasis	Lupus	Rothmund-Thomson syndrome	Acrodermatitis chronicum atrophicans
Lymphoma	DM	Bloom syndrome Dyskeratosis congenita Fanconi syndrome XP Werner syndrome Kindler syndrome (congenital acral blisters, dystrophy, photosensitivity, oral erosions)	Lyme disease

TABLE 12–3
DERMATOSES OF PREGNANCY

Disease	Trimester	Clinical Manifestations (on Fetus)	Treatment (for Mother)
Rubella	First	Cataracts, congenital heart defects, deafness	
Parvovirus B19	First 20 weeks	Hydrops fetalis	
Early syphilis	20–40 weeks	40% die, 40% infected	PCN G
PUPPP	Third	Elevated risk: primigravida, twins; spares umbilicus	
Herpes gestationis	Second to third	5% babies with bullae; may flare after delivery	Steroids
Cholestasis (elevated bilirubin)	Third	Pruritus	
Impetigo herpetiformis	Third	Fetal death, hypocalcemia	
VZV	1st 20 weeks	1–2% hypoplastic limbs, CNS/ocular disease, scars	IV acyclovir
VZV	25–36 weeks	Infantile zoster 1%	IVIg may help
VZV	5 days before + 2 days after delivery	1% severe neonatal zoster (one-third die)	IVIg + IV acyclovir

ABBREVIATIONS: PUPPP = pruritic urticarial papules and plaques of pregnancy; VZV = varicella zoster virus.

TABLE 12–4
DIFFERENTIAL DIAGNOSIS OF PSEUDOAINHUM

Hereditary	Nonhereditary
Erythropoietic protoporphyria	Syringomyelia
Ehlers-Danlos syndrome	Scleroderma
Pachyonychia congenita	Pityriasis rubra pilaris
Mal de Meleda	Psoriasis
Vohwinkel PPK*	Ergot poisoning
Olmstead syndrome	Leprosy

*Palmoplantar keratoderma.

DIFFERENTIAL DIAGNOSIS OF SADDLE-NOSE DEFORMITY

Congenital	Idiopathic	Infectious
Congenital syphilis	Wegener granulomatosis	Lepromatous leprosy
Congenital rubella	Relapsing polychondritis	Leishmaniasis
Anhidrotic ectodermal dysplasia ("sad facies" associated with hypothermia)		
Other		
Hurler syndrome		

DIFFERENTIAL DIAGNOSIS OF SCLERODERMA

The most common cause of death in scleroderma is renal or cardiac failure; use captopril to treat.

"Sclero"	"Eosinophil"	Genetic	Metabolic
Scleredema	Eosinophilic fasciitis	Progeria	PCT
Scleromyxedema (GI symptom = dysphagia)	Eosinophilia myalgia syndrome (L-tryptophan, rapeseed oil)	Werner syndrome	Diabetic stiff skin

Immunologic	Chemical	Environmental	Neoplastic
Chronic GVH (sclerodermoid)	Polyvinyl chloride	Radiation	Scirrhous breast cancer (diffuse infiltration, secondary metastases)
Human adjuvant disease	Bleomycin Vincristine Vitamin K	Silicosis	

TABLE 12–5
SENSITIVITY AND SPECIFICITY

	Disease Present[a,c]	Disease Absent[b,d]	
Test positive	True positive (TP)	False positive (FP)	All positive (AP)
Test negative	False negative (FN)	True negative (TN)	All negative (AN)
	With disease (WD)	Without disease (WOD)	Total sample size

[a] Sensitivity = TP/AP
[b] Positive predictive value = TP/WD
[c] Specificity = TN/AN
[d] Negative predictive value =TN/WOD

SUNSCREENS

Contact allergens include

- PABA
- Benzophenones
- Cinnamates
- Methoxydibenzoylmethane (Parsol 1789)

TABLE 12–6
TYPES OF SUNSCREENS[a]

Benzophenones		
Cinnamates, Salicylates, PABA	Anthralinates	Dibenzoyl Methanes
290 ← UVB → 320	320 ← UVA2 → 340	340 ← UVA1 → 400

[a] Physical blockers include titanium dioxide and zinc oxide.

DIFFERENTIAL DIAGNOSIS OF SUPPURATIVE LYMPHADENITIS

- Scrofuloderma
- Cat-scratch disease
- Paracoccidioido-mycosis
- Plague
- Rat-bite fever
- Atypical mycobacteria
- Coccidioidomycosis
- Actinomycosis
- Dental sinus (get dental x-ray)
- Acne conglobata
- Tularemia
- Histoplasmosis
- Nocardiosis
- Hidradenitis suppurativa
- Syphilis

DIFFERENTIAL DIAGNOSIS OF ULCERS

Mnemonic: Vitamin C

Vasculitis
Infection
Trauma
Autoimmune
Medications
Idiopathic
Neoplasm
Congenital

DIFFERENTIAL DIAGNOSIS OF DARK URINE

Hepatic erythropoeitic porphyria (port wine)
Erythropoeitic porphyria (Gunther) (port wine)
Acute intermittent porphyria (during attack)
Alkaptonuria
Rhabdomyolysis

DIFFERENTIAL DIAGNOSIS OF VERRUCOUS LESION

- Halogenoderma (peripheral yellow pustules)
- Tuberculosis verrucosa cutis
- Verrucous carcinomas
- Chromomycosis
- Paracoccidioidomycosis
- Blastomycosis (peripheral yellow pustules)
- SCC

TABLE 12–7
WOOD'S LIGHT EXAMINATION[a]

Disease	Etiology	Fluorescent Agent	Fluorescent Color	Regular Light
Tinea capitis	*Microsporum audouini* or *Microsporum canis*	Pteridine	Bright yellow-green	
Erythrasma	*Corynebacterium minutissimum*	Coproporphyrin III	Coral red	
Pseudomonas (interdigital)	*Pseudomonas aeruginosa*	Pyoverdin = fluorescein	Bright aqua-green to white-green	Pyocyanin = green
Porphyria cutanea tarda	Uroporphyrin decarboxylase deficiency	Uroporphyrins	Pink-orange	
Trichomycosis axillaris	*Corynebacterium tenuis*		Orange	
Superficial white onychomycosis	*Trichophyton mentagrophytes*		Bright white	White

[a] Mercury lamp with nickel oxide filter; $\lambda = 365$ nm.

TABLE 12–8
DIAGNOSES AND ASSOCIATIONS

Lesion	Associated Disease
Basal cell carcinoma	Bazex-Dupre-Christol: atrophoderma vermiculatum, BCCs, hypohidrosis, hypotrichosis
Basal cell carcinoma	Rombo syndrome (BCCs, milia, atrophoderma vermiculatum, acral cyanosis, hypotrichosis)
Clear cell syringoma	Diabetes
Cylindroma	Ancell-Spiegler or Brook-Fordyce syndromes (multiple trichoepitheliomas + multiple cylindromas)
Cylindroma	Rasmussen syndrome (multiple trichoepitheliomas + multiple cylindromas + milia)
Cylindroma	Parotid gland tumors
Cylindroma	Eccrine spiradenoma
Dermatofibromas (multiple)	Systemic lupus, HIV
Desmoplastic trichoepithelioma	Melanocytic nevus (admixed in 15% of cases)
Eccrine syringofibroadenoma	Schopf syndrome=hidrocystomas, hypotrichosis, hypodontia, anonychia
Fibrofolliculomas	Birt-Hogg-Dube syndrome
Follicular spicules on nose	Multiple myeloma
Hemorrhagic nodules	Chronic meningococcemia
Heliotrope eruption	Dermatomyositis, hyperaldosteronism
Hidrocystomas	Schopf syndrome=eccrine syringofibroadenomas, hypotrichosis, hypodontia, anonychia
Keratoacanthomas, eruptive	Immunosuppression, systemic lupus
Koplik spots	Measles: altered sebaceous glands on mucosa, not on palate
Nevus sebaceous	BCC, syringocystadenoma, trichoblastoma; Schimmel-Penning syndrome: deafness, mental retardation, seizures, colobomas, lipodermoids
Nevus comedonicus	Alagille syndrome (arteriohepatic dysplasia)
Osteolysis in clavicle, arthritis	Acne fulminans
Pilomatricoma	Myotonic dystrophy, baldness, Raynaud
Pilomatricoma	Rubinstein-Taybi syndrome
Pilomatricoma	β-catenin overexpressed

TABLE 12–8
DIAGNOSES AND ASSOCIATIONS (*Continued*)

Lesion	Associated Disease
Pilomatrical changes in EIC	Gardner syndrome
Pustule, malignant	Anthrax (Woolsorter disease)
Psammomatous melanotic schwannoma	Carney complex
Sclerotic fibroma	Cowden syndrome
Sebaceous adenoma and carcinoma	Muir-Torre syndrome (colon cancer), cancer family syndrome
Syringoma	Down syndrome
Syringomas (eruptive)	With milia + atrophoderma vermiculatum = Nicolau-Balus syndrome
Trichodiscomas	Birt-Hogg-Dube syndrome
Trichoepitheliomas	Rombo syndrome (BCCs, milia, atrophoderma vermiculatum, acral cyanosis, hypotrichosis)
Trichoepitheliomas	Ancell-Spiegler or Brook-Fordyce syndromes (multiple trichoepitheliomas + multiple cylindromas)
Trichoepitheliomas	Rasmussen syndrome (multiple trichoepitheliomas + multiple cylindromas + milia)
Trichilemmoma	Cowden syndrome (breast cancer, thyroid cancer, hamartomas), Bannayan-Riley-Ruvalcaba syndrome (venous/lymph malformations, macrocephaly, lipoangiomatosis, spotted penis pigmentation, intestinal polyps)

TABLE 12–9
DIAGNOSES AND ASSOCIATIONS

Diagnosis	Associated Disease
Alopecia areata	Hashimoto thyroiditis, pernicious anemia, Addison disease, vitiligo
Angiosarcoma	After lymphectomy for carcinoma: Stuart-Treves syndrome (arm); Kettle syndrome (leg)
Bazex syndrome	Violaceous acral sites, palmoplantar keratoderma, dystrophy = upper aerodigestive malignancy
Birt-Hogg-Dube syndrome	Renal carcinoma, colonic polyps
Chronic mucocutaneous candidiasis	Adult: yhymoma, children (usually < age 6): hypoparathyroidism (endocrinopathy)
Dermatitis herpetiformis	Celiac disease, thyroid disease, lymphoma, exacerbated by NSAIDs
Dermatomyositis, juvenile	Calcification, vasculitis of muscles + GI tract, arthritis, hypertrichosis, lipoatrophy, gingival telangiectasia
Dermatomyositis, adult	Ovarian, stomach, and lung cancer
Dupuytren (hand)/Ledderhose (foot) disease	Alcoholic cirrhosis, diabetes, chronic epilepsy
Epidermolysis bullosa acquisita	Inflammatory bowel disease
Erythema gyratum repens	Lung or breast cancer, hypertrichosis lanuginosa acquisita
Erythema marginatum	Rheumatic fever
Frey syndrome	Gustatory sweating on face that occurs after neck surgery
Granulomatous slack skin	Hodgkin lymphoma
Hair collar sign	Encephalocele or meningioma
Heparin-induced necrosis	Antibodies to heparin
Hypertrichosis lanuginosa acquisita	"Malignant down" associated with lung or colon malignancy
Infective dermatitis	HTLV-1, recurrent seborrheic rash

TABLE 12–9
DIAGNOSES AND ASSOCIATIONS (*Continued*)

Diagnosis	Associated Disease
Inflammatory bowel disease	Pyostomatitis vegetans, EBA, pyoderma gangrenosum (ulcerative colitis)
Kaposiform hemangioenothelioma	Kasabach-Merritt syndrome (mortality 30%), usually retroperitoneal
Lipodystrophy, partial	C3 deficiency, glomerulonephritis
Madelung disease (horse-collar sign)	Bilateral symmetrical lipomatosis associated with upper respiratory tract cancer
Malum perforans	Neurotophic ulcer on the sole caused by decreased sensation in leprosy, diabetes, tabes dorsalis
Merkel cell carcinoma	Multiple SCCs, BCCs, lymphoma, malignant melanoma
Migratory thrombophlebitis (Trousseau)	Pancreatic cancer
Morphea of the breast	Supervoltage radiation therapy
Necrolytic migratory erythema	Glucagonoma of pancreatic α-islet cell tumor
Oral lichen planus	Grinspan syndrome: oral lichen planus, hypertension, diabetes mellitus
Pachydermyperiostosis (acquired)	Bronchogenic carcinoma
Pemphigus vulgaris	Myasthenia gravis, thymoma
Peyronie disease (penis)	Firm palmar nodules proximal to fourth finger; caused by fibromatosis of palmar aponeurosis
Pityriasis rotunda	Hepatocellular cancer
Protein S deficiency	Behcet syndrome, cardiac manifestations
Purpura fulminans	Protein C deficiency
Pyogenic granuloma	Pregnancy, isotretinoin (Accutane)
Rowell syndrome	Lupus and erythema muliforme concomitantly
Seborrheic keratoses (eruptive) = Leser-Trelat	Precedes malignancy, stomach cancer, osteogenic sarcoma

Sister Mary Joseph nodule (periumbilical nodule)	Stomach, colon, ovarian, or pancreatic cancer. Also endometriosis, urachal duct cyst, omphalocele, and Meckel diverticulum
Steatocystoma	Steatocystoma multiplex, pachyonychia congenita II (Jackson-Lawler syndrome)
Sweet syndrome	AML, ulcerative colitis, other heme malignancy
Thrombophlebitis of chest wall (Mondor disease)	Breast carcinoma
Tripe palms (acanthosis nigricans)	Stomach or lung cancer
Tufted angioma	Kasabach-Merritt syndrome, usually retroperitoneal
Vitiligo	Thyroid disease, autoimmune disease, APECED syndrome, psoriasis + HIV, Addison disease
Warfarin (Coumadin) necrosis	Protein C deficiency (occasional protein S or antithrombin III deficiency)

TABLE 12–10
DIAGNOSES AND ASSOCIATIONS

Lesion	Clinical or Pathologic Finding
Accessory tragus	Numerous vellous hairs, subcutaenous fat, occasional cartilage; wattle located on neck; origin: first branchial arch
Accessory digit	Acral, fibrous stroma, nerves
Accessory nipple	Invaginated pilosebaceous unit, underlying glands + muscle; "milk line"
Adenoid cystic carcinoma/eccrine epithelioma	Scalp; perineural invasion; similar to microcystic adnexal carcinoma
Annular elastolytic granuloma	Elastophagocytolysis on pathology
Atrophoderma of Pasini and Perini	Most common location: back
Becker nevus	Testosterone receptors
Café-au-lait (CAL) macules	Neonate: buttocks; infant: trunk
Cellular blue nevus	Most common location: buttocks
Cheilitis glandularis	Inflammatory cells around salivary glands
Chloracne	Retroauricular location
Chondroid syringoma (mixed tumor)	Most common is head + neck; pseudocartilaginous, lace-like patterns of pale blue cells, ducts, mucinous stroma
CMV infection	Enlarged endothelial cells
Cylindroma	Jigsaw puzzle; scalp
Dermal duct tumor	Monomorphic big blue balls (like poroma) with small ducts only in dermis (see hidroacanthoma)
Dermatofibroma sarcoma protuberans	Most common locations: thigh, trunk
Desmoplastic trichoepithelioma	Depressed center; syringoma-like with horn cysts, fibrovascular stroma, focal calcification
Diabetic dermopathy	PAS+ fibrillar material in thickened vessel walls, lamina lucida split
Dysplastic nevus	VFIB: vascularity, fibrosis, intercellular bridging
Eccrine hidrocystoma	Seasonal variation, eyelids
Eccrine poroma	Monomorphic blue tumor with small ducts extending from epidermis (dermal duct, hidroacanthoma)

Eccrine spiradenoma	Painful; overlying skin blue; blue balls in dermis with ductal differentiation, alveolar pattern
Eccrine syringofibroadenoma	Anastomosing epithelial strands surrounded by fibrous stroma; "hamburger" meat appearance
Elastosis perforans serpiginosa	Narrow channel with "raveled wool" appearance; "bramblebush" in drug-induced type; second decade
Erythema ab igne	Elastosis
Extramammary Paget disease	Underpants erythema (redness of legs)
Fibrofolliculoma	Cystically dilated follicle, proliferation of outer root sheath epithelium + perifollicular fibrosis
Giant cell tumor of tendon sheath	Osteoclast-like giant cells, lipophages, siderophages, flexor surfaces, 25% recurrence
Granular cell tumor	Tongue
Hidradenoma papilliferum	Vulva; epithelial papillae, usually no epidermal component
Hidroacanthoma simplex	Acanthotic epidermis, intraepidermal monomorphic blue cells with small ducts (see poroma, dermal duct)
Hypopigmented CTCL	Younger, darker skinned patients, good prognosis (do not go beyond stage 1)
Idiopathic plantar hidradenitis	Children, self-limited
Juvenile plantar dermatosis	Eczematous eruption on both soles; shiny appearance
Kaposi sarcoma	Plasma cells; spindle endothelial cells trapping RBCs
Keratolysis exfoliativa	Idiopathic peeling of hands and feet
Kyrle disease/perforating folliculitis	Widened follicle with plug and impending rupture/perforation; patients 20–60 years old, diabetics
Lanugo hair	Most common site is face
Lupus panniculitis	Plasma cells; lymphoid follicles waxy pink lipodegeneration; treat with hydroxychloroquine (Plaquenil)
Malignant chondroid syringoma	Metastatic lesions may have minimal chondroid component
Malignant fibrohistiocytoma	Most common location is thigh
Mastocytoma, solitary	Majority on dorsal hand, involute by age 10
Microcystic adnexal carcinoma	Upper lip, high local recurrence; appears like a deep invasive syringoma
Mucinous adenocarcinoma	Pools of mucin, suspended islands of tumor cells
Necrobiosis lipoidica	Plasma cells; "layer cake" of necrobiosis and inflammation deep into fat
Necrobiotic xanthogranuloma	Primary biliary cirrhosis, paraproteinemia, multiple myeloma, IgG-kappa chain

TABLE 12–10
DIAGNOSES AND ASSOCIATIONS (*Continued*)

Lesion	Clinical or Pathologic Finding
Neurofibromas	Mast cells, comma-shaped nuclei
Nevus sebaceous	Apocrine glands notable in adult biopsy; infant biopsy: sebaceous glands at epidermis
Nodular hidradenoma/eccrine acrospiroma	Blue balls in dermis with cystic degeneration, clear cell change
Papillary adenocarcinoma (aggressive digital)	Digits, high local recurrence
Papillary eccrine adenoma	Blacks, females, legs; dermal cystically dilated ducts with epithelial processes
Palmoplantar pustulosis	Bilateral clavicular sterile osteomyelitis, "lakes of pus"
Parakeratosis pustulosis	Pediatric, thumb or index finger, probable variant of psoriasis, resolves at puberty
Pilar (trichilemmal) cyst	Basal cell layer, squamous layer, no granular layer, homogenous eosinophilic contents
Pilar sheath acanthoma	Upper lip, widened pore with invagination
Pilomatricoma	Shadow cells, blue cells, hard nodule, younger patients, calcification
Porocarcinoma	Cutaneous (epidermotropic mets)
Proliferating trichilemmal tumor	Scalp, SCC-like, no shadow cells, lobular growth
Pseudolymphoma	Phenytoin (Dilantin)
Reacting perforating collagenosis	Broad superficial cup-like perforation with red-blue material; seen in children
SAPHO syndrome	Synovitis, acne, pustulosis, hyperostosis, osteitis
Sebaceous carcinoma	Eyelids; in situ, pagetoid spread
Sinus histiocytosis (Rosai-Dorfman)	Emperipolesis = intact lymphocytes within histiocytes
Sjögren lesions	Inflammatory cells around salivary glands + lymphocytic vasculitis
Steatocystoma	Corrugated lining, sebaceous glands
Syringocystadenoma papilliferum	Invagination from epidermis, double layered epithelial papillae, apocrine glands; plasma cells
Syringoma	Females, eyelids, possibly hormonally controlled

Telangiectasia macularis eruptiva perstans (TMEP)	Negative Darier sign, peptic ulcer disease, bone lesions
Traction alopecia, trichotillomania	Melanin casts are clumps of melanin in follicle
Trichoadenoma	Numerous dermal keratin cysts, fibrovascular stroma
Trichodiscoma	Raised papule, lateral collarette, fibrous proliferation in dermis
Trichoepithelioma	Palisaded blue balls with horn cysts, papillary mesenchymal bodies, no retraction
Trichofolliculoma	Tuft of hair; well-developed dilated follicle surrounded by multiple smaller follicles
Trichilemmoma	Warty, acanthosis with clear glycogen filled keratinocytes
Tumor of the follicular infundibulum	Plate-like growth of follicular epithelium
Vellous hair cyst	Thin-walled, many vellous hairs
Verruciform xanthoma	Oral cavity
Xanthomas	Doubly refractile lipids
Zoon balanitis	Smooth red-orange plaque with cayenne pepper appearance; plasma cells

INDEX

Note: Page numbers followed by *f* indicate figures; those followed by *t* indicate tables.

D

T